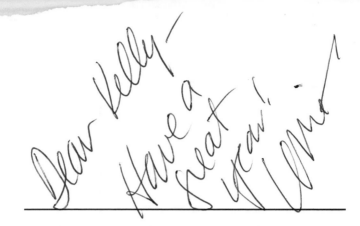

Why Can't I Lose Weight Cookbook

Healthy, delicious recipes for
successful, permanent weight loss

by

Lorrie Medford, C.N.

P9-CBT-638

LDN Publishing
P.O. Box 54007
Tulsa, Oklahoma 74155

WHY CAN'T I LOSE WEIGHT COOKBOOK
Healthy, delicious recipes for
successful permanent weight loss
Copy © 2001 Lorrie Medford, CN
LDN Publishing
PO Box 54007
Tulsa, OK 74155

Library of Congress Cataloging-in-Publishing Data

Medford, Lorrie, 1949

> *Why Can't I Lose Weight Cookbook*
> Lorrie Medford, C.N.
> International Standard Book Number: 0-9676419-1-8
> 1. Cookbook. 2. Weight loss 3. Nutrition. 4. Health. 5. Title

NOTE: This program is designed for healthy adults. If you have special health needs such as chronic disease, diabetes, heart conditions, pregnancy or are a lactating woman, or have a medical condition that requires medical attention, consult your health care provider for assistance and advice before beginning this program.

Printed in the United States of America

10 9 8 7 6 5 4 3 2 1 First U. S. Edition

(For ordering information, refer to the back pages of this book.)

Dedication

This book is dedicated to my clients who have waited patiently for these recipes. I pray God's abundant grace, love and healing for you, all the days of your lives.

Contents

Part Five: Appendices

Foreword

This book not only contains practical, satisfying and delicious recipes, but it's also an incredible wealth of information on nutrition, with lots of tips on the how-to's, whys, and benefits of eating wholesome foods. I love the way the recipes are so balanced and no artificial sweeteners or flavorings are used.

It is obvious to me that Lorrie truly lives this way of healthy eating which makes it easy for a novice to adapt her favorite recipes as a lifestyle.

This book has been written from a heart that cares for people, with the understanding that everyone loves to eat good, tasty, hearty foods.

God bless you, Lorrie—you have not only given us your heart and years of research for wholesome foods, but also shown us that we can be healthy and lose weight safely, too!

This book will inspire you to cook and eat healthy for life.

—PAT HARRISON
PRESIDENT
FAITH CHRISTIAN FELLOWSHIP INT'L
TULSA, OKLAHOMA

Acknowledgements

I especially want to acknowledge several people who read my manuscript thoroughly and made valuable comments throughout: Thanks to Katrina Raynor, Susan Brooks, and Michelle Young. Thanks for all of your excellent feedback and encouragement to publish this cookbook. Thanks, Katrina, for our delightful evening of experimenting with some of these recipes. Thanks, Michelle, for hosting a dinner party to try several of my recipes. We were all wonderfully stuffed! And Susan, thanks for trying so many of my recipes and making great suggestions for improving them. I loved your comments!

I really appreciate and thank Carol Enders and Vicky Musser who both tried several new recipes on their family and friends. Your results determined what recipes might be included in this book.

Thanks to my assistants, Anne Spears, Carolyn Clark, and Jackie Charest. You are all a blessing and I thank you for your help in putting this cookbook together.

Special thanks to Julianna Grace for all of your hard work editing, writing the index, and just general support and encouragement! So often I thought, "I don't know what I would have done without Julianna." And your Austrailian perspective was most welcome!

Many thanks to my talented graphic designer, Brandon Sensintaffar for the cover design work.

Thanks to my friend, Dr. Jeff Magee, who is always so gracious and willing to help me with the many numerous decisions regarding book publishing.

Thanks to Lindsay Roberts for your encouragement to publish this cookbook, and especially for your comments about which chapters to include. I appreciate you, your passion for nutrition, and your passion for the things of God.

Special thanks to Pat Harrison. Thanks for taking time out of your busy schedule to write a foreword for this book. I am grateful for your encouragement and support. You are always an inspiration to me.

Most of all, I thank God, without Whom I am nothing, and I can do nothing.

About the Author

Author and motivational speaker, Lorrie Medford has a BA in Communications and is a licensed Certified Nutritionist from The American Health Science University. She also holds certification as a personal trainer from ISSA (International Sports Science Association). She serves on the Board of Directors for the Society of Certified Nutritionists, and is a member of the Oklahoma Speakers Association. Lorrie is also on the Advisory Board for Standard Process, Inc.

In addition to writing this cookbook, Lorrie has also written a motivation book, *Why Can't I Stay Motivated?*, and a weight-loss book, *Why Can't I Lose Weight?* A health researcher and journalist, Lorrie has studied nutrition, whole-foods cooking, herbs, health, fitness, and motivation for more than 20 years. Lorrie taught her weight-loss class at a local junior college and within her own business for more than 10 years, and has taught natural food cooking classes in Spokane, Washington and Tulsa, Oklahoma for more than 5 years.

She shares her knowledge not only in this book, but also in her seminars, and through her nutritional consultation practice, *Life Design Nutrition* in Tulsa, Oklahoma.

Lorrie is uniquely qualified to write about health and fitness. She knows what it's like to be a *cranky calorie counter* obsessed with foods, dieting, and striving to be thin. After struggling with her weight for many years, Lorrie lost more than 35 pounds and has kept it off for more than sixteen years by following the ideas presented in this book.

Lorrie has a rich history of community involvement teaching nutrition, and is a sought-after speaker for civic groups, churches, hospitals, and wellness organizations.

We Can All Win the "No-Belly" Prize!

The other day, a friend of mine said he was eating a homemade turnover. Surprised at his ability to bake, I asked where he found the recipe. He replied, "Oh, I bought it at the store, but I baked it in the oven myself!

People's idea of cooking today combines boiling water for frozen entrees, heating on the stove or zapping in the microwave! We have so many appliances in our kitchen, if we used them all, we'd have a power shortage. Food is so instant, that we even have instant heart burn!

We've come a long way from the days of baking every-thing from scratch and spending hours in the kitchen. Unfortunately, we've also come a long way from eating foods that really help us burn fat and lose weight. Only about nine percent of Americans eat their five servings of fruits and veg-etables. Currently, nearly 50% of our population struggles with weight loss. Everywhere we look, the growing body of research shows that the foods we eat effect our weight, health, appearance, attitude, and longevity. We can lose weight much easier if we eat foods that encourage weight loss.

How I Got Started

Understanding my background explains my approach with this cookbook. In the early 1970s, my two sisters and I started changing our diets when our father was diagnosed with lung cancer. We read everything we could find about eating healthier. We noticed that when he ate well, his condition improved. Although natural measures were too late, his death motivated me to further study.

From that time, I took many nutrition courses and read everything I could find about health and nutrition. During one year, I flew to both California and Boston to learn how to cook and bake from scratch using whole natural foods. Back in Seattle, I attended several more cooking classes from various teachers. I wanted to develop recipes that were not only healthy, but tasted good as well. In April 1977 I began teaching cooking classes which I taught regularly for the next three years at various churches and holistic health centers throughout Spokane, Washington.

Pleasingly Plump

In Spokane, I offered "Monday Night Dinners" for a year where people could come to my home and enjoy a delicious homemade meal. For two hours, my house was filled with the aroma of freshly-baked whole-grain bread. However, at the end of the evening my tummy was also filled with whole-grain bread! My compulsive overeating habit lead me to become a cranky calorie counter. In spite of the fact that I was eating healthier foods, I was gaining more and more weight.

As I continued studying nutrition and the effect of food on weight gain, my pudgy pounds began to come off and stay off. My attitude towards weight loss was changing from a "dieting mentality" to the understanding that weight loss was a health issue and it had to be a lifestyle change. Along the way, I made extensive studies of motivation.

Winning the Prize

I finally lost more than 35 pounds, which I have kept off for more than 17 years. In 1989, I started teaching a course in Tulsa, Oklahoma on weight loss from a health perspective which I taught for nearly 10 years. This class allowed me to teach what I had learned about how to lose weight easily and safely with healthy foods. After teaching people about the benefits of whole natural foods on weight loss, they now wanted to know how to cook! So I again taught cooking classes every month for a year at a local health food store.

I've seen more than 3,000 clients as a practicing Certified Nutritionist and now have a better understanding of what people need for health and weight loss. Combining these recipes with my philosophy helps people lose weight safely.

Make It a Lifestyle

In my first book, *Why Can't I Lose Weight?*, I said that to lose weight permanently requires two things:

1. Discover what's been hindering your weight loss.

2. Make it a lifestyle this time. A healthy diet, along with healthy eating patterns, needs to become a lifestyle—a way of life.

Designing your life for health and weight loss means planning healthy meals. So in this book, I'll help you: 1) Make time for meal planning, shopping and preparing food; and 2) Make recipes that are tasty, easy to make, and fairly quick. (For even more help with designing your life, see my second book, *Why Can't I Stay Motivated?*)

Where Do You Need Help?

Broken into five parts, this book presents ideas for planning and preparing foods for successful weight loss. Packed with tips on quick snacks, healthy meals and meal planning, this book shows you what to do, why to do it, and how to do it.

Part One gives my philosophy about weight loss and why I recommend the foods in this cookbook.

Part Two is about designing your kitchen for weight loss. It gives you an extensive shopping list, and helpful tips for using herbs and spices.

Part Three tells you how wonderful vegetables are for health and weight loss as well as meal planning, tips for quick meals, and how to eat out and still stay slim.

Part Four contains easy, healthy recipes including beverages, salad dressings, salads, vegetable entrees, soups and chilies, chicken, fish, egg dishes, whole grains, pasta, muffins, whole-grain breads and natural desserts.

Part Five contains additional information including cooking techniques, helpful utensils, weights and measures, sugar substitutes, and a glossary of herbs and spices, beans and grains.

You Can Cook Healthy

Everyone of us eat about 21 meals every week. These meals determine our health and weight. With just a few minutes of planning every week, you can put together healthy meals that will move you to your health goals. My desire is that this book will help you do just that.

Now you too can enjoy greater health by delicious, healthy cooking!

PART ONE

The Life Design Philosophy of Weight Loss

Chapter One

Why Foods Make Us Fat

Browsing through your local bookstore, you'll see dozens of books on diets. Some books advocate a high-protein, low-carbohydrate diet, while others tell you to eat a high-carbohydrate, low-protein diet. Still others advocate a high-fiber diet or vegetarian diet. Then there are blood or body type diets. Even if you've only read one or two of these books, you may be confused when the authors start to contradict each other!

As a practicing Certified Nutritionist, I can see as many as 30 follow-up appointments a day, and I've interviewed thousands of people in the last 15 years. I've met people who eat only twice a day and keep their weight normal. I've had clients who eat moderate protein and are healthy and losing weight. I've worked with body builders and vegetarians. I've had a first-hand opportunity to see what really works and where people have problems.

What Really Makes Us Fat?

In my first book, *Why Can't I Lose Weight?*, I explained in detail how we can get fat from the foods we eat. Here, let's just review the three ways our standard American diet is making us fat.

1. How Sugar Makes Us Fat

Have you seen the typical American diet lately? Take a peak at the office break room, and see what's there. What's quick, tasty, and easy to take to the office for a reward? How about a birthday? Or an anniversary? Sweets! Pick from cakes, cookies, donuts, or sweet breads. It's American, it's tradition, and it's settled! We reward ourselves with sweets, usually sweetened with refined white sugar. You know, the "pure" stuff.

Eating sugar or refined carbohydrates raises the amount of circulating insulin which is the fat-storing, hunger hormone. Eating protein raises the circulating glucagon, which is the anti-hunger, fat-burning hormone. While I am not an advocate of an all-protein diet, I do recommend that people eat at least 2-3 servings of protein a day, especially for weight loss. Lowering your sugar intake is crucial for effective weight loss.

Most of my clients report that eating a balanced meal of protein, vegetables and starch is so satisfying that they don't go looking for something else to eat afterwards. (However, for those who want to slowly wean off desserts, I have included a few healthy desserts in this cookbook.)

2. How Carbohydrates Make Us Fat

Processed carbohydrates are foods made from white flour such as white bagels, cookies, cakes and pasta. Processed carbohydrates can make us fat because they act like a sugar in the body.

Since the Government's new Food Pyramid which recommended from 6 to 11 daily servings of carbohydrates, half the population is overweight. Many people ate a "low-fat" diet that only complicated their weight-loss problem because they cut out the fat and ate more sugar and carbohydrates. Unfortunately, many of the nutritional guidelines we follow are given to us by the food industries that make processed foods, not by clinical nutritionists or scientists.

Clients often ask: "Do we have to give up pasta, bread, and potatoes to lose weight?" There are two ways to eat carbohydrates and still lose weight. One is to cut down the total number of daily servings, and another is to eat carbohydrates that are high in fiber, like slow-cooking oatmeal, or real whole-grain bread—not the white stuff that has been colored with caramel coloring. The recipes in this book include whole-grain products such as breads, muffins and pasta which you can eat moderately.

3. How Fats Make Us Fat

Obviously, too much of any fat can make us fat. That's why we all originally cut out fat. But when we cut fat out of our diets, the unfortunate thing is that we cut out the *good* fats as well as the bad. Bad fats are processed fats. They can put weight on because they are so indigestible. These bad fats include vegetable oils which were damaged in processing with high temperatures or chemicals, and hydrogenated and partially-hydrogenated oils, such as margarine. In the hydrogenation process, hydrogen molecules are added to a good vegetable oil which damages the fat and also makes it saturated. These damaged fats are linked to free radical damage, heart disease and cancer. You won't find any recipes in this cookbook which use margarine or deep-frying methods.

What about all of these hydrogenated fake butters that don't melt and taste awful? Butter is better. Hydrogenation is great for preserving the food, but not for preserving us. If the food you are considering buying starts with the phrase, "I can't believe it's...." you probably can believe that it's not a real food. (I can't believe that people still buy these foods!)

Good Fats Burn Fat

Going fat-free is no fun! Like some of my clients, when I tried to not eat fat, I found myself squeezing Haagen-daz in my otherwise healthy diet. God made us to need and enjoy good fat.

20

Did you know that adding good fat to your diet can help you burn fat? In my weight-loss book, I quoted Udo Urasmus who gave several tablespoons of flaxseed oil to one of his clients and she lost 50 pounds! Adding one tablespoon of flaxseed oil to your diet daily can help you burn fat. Flaxseed is a wonderful fat which helps every part of your body, especially your brain, immune system, hormones, hair, skin and nails. These oils are clinically proven to also lower cholesterol and help prevent cancer. (I've included a section on oils on pages 109-111.) While you will find a variety of fats throughout these recipes, I have also given low-fat recipes and low-fat cooking methods, too.

Proteins are vital for health and fat-burning, unless you eat high-fat, processed meats such as sausage and bacon. The key to eating protein is to balance it with lots of fresh fruits and vegetables, small amounts of carbohydrates and good fats.

An extensive meal plan and serving sizes are given in chapter five.

PART TWO

The Life Design Kitchen

Chapter Two

Healthy Shopping

Shopping in a supermarket can be an overwhelming experience. Amy, another client recently said, "I went to the grocery store with a conscious decision to read the labels and buy healthy foods. But thirty minutes later, I just gave up and threw whatever I saw in the basket! It's too overwhelming to read every label. Even then, you don't know what you're getting!"

Find Healthier Options

This is a common reaction! Americans are so accustomed to buying and eating processed foods that we find it awkward and even difficult to change. How can you quickly spot healthy foods among so many processed ones?

Throughout the years, I have accompanied clients as they shopped in their local grocery stores teaching them to sort through the thousands of packaged foods and make smarter selections. I walked one of my clients through a national chain supermarket. Come through the aisles with us as we look for foods to make healthy meals for weight loss.

Fruits

Here we are at the produce aisles looking at whole fresh fruits. Fresh produce is packed with vitamins, minerals and enzymes, all vital for healthy weight loss.

It's best to eat fruits alone, in their raw, fresh state. Many people like to make a meal of a fruit salad, or eat them as snacks. Either way, most people need some protein for breakfast too, so add some raw nuts like almonds or cashews (10 per day). Canned fruit has no enzymes and is often loaded with extra sugar, so frozen is preferred over canned. If you do use canned fruit, buy the fruit packed in light syrup, or with no added sugar.

Vegetables

Also in the produce section, you'll find all the fresh vegetables. You can eat vegetables raw, lightly steamed, in a salad, baked or stir-fried, with a little bit of olive oil or butter. Herbal seasonings add some flavor.

As for salads, look for the dark-green leafy vegetables like romaine and green leaf lettuce. Forget the iceberg lettuce since it's low in nutrition. Your local grocery store and health food store both carry ready-to-eat salad mixes.

Read a label or two on canned vegetables and you'll see that sugar is commonly added. Ditch the canned vegetables, and for convenience, get frozen vegetables. The trick here is to get them without all those extra fatty sauces, sugar or chemicals.

Fruits	**Vegetables**
Apples	Alfalfa sprouts
Applesauce, unsweetened	Artichokes
Apricots	Asparagus
Bananas	Bamboo Shoots
Berries:	Beets/beet greens
Blackberry	Bok Choy
Blueberry	Bell Peppers
Boysenberry	Broccoli
Cranberry	Brussels Sprouts
Elderberry	Cabbage
Gooseberry	Carrots
Raspberry	Cauliflower

25

Fruits

Strawberry
Cherries
Dates
Figs, dried or fresh
Grapefruit
Grapes, red or green
Kiwi fruit
Lemons
Limes
Mandarin oranges
Mango
Melons:
  Cantaloupe
  Cassava
  Honeydew
  Watermelon
Nectarines
Oranges/Tangerines
Papaya
Passion fruit
Peaches
Pears
Pineapple
Plums
Prunes
Raisins
Watermelon
Fruit leather (100% fruit)

Vegetables

Celery
Corn on the cob
Cucumbers
Endive
Green Beans
Leeks
Lettuce: red, green leaf
Mushrooms
Onions, red, white
Peppers, bell, cherry, red
Potatoes, red, white
Radishes
Romaine Lettuce
Snow Peas
Spaghetti Squash
Spinach
Squashes
Sugar Snap Peas
Tomatoes
Turnips
Yams
Watercress
Zucchini

Salad Dressings

Many people skip the French Fries, but they load their salads with hydrogenated salad dressings or mayonnaise. Check out the labels on many of the grocery salad dressings and you'll also find sugar or hydrogenated oils! You are

allowed *some* fat in your diet. Here are some healthier suggestions.   Use extra virgin olive oil or flaxseed oil and lemon
juice for your salads. Get a healthy (non-hydrogenated) salad
dressing, like Cardinis. Or go to your local health food store
and buy "healthy" fat-free salad dressings like these.

> Tree of Life low-fat dressings
> Spectrum dressings (Low-fat Southwest Caesar, Honey Dijon, etc.)
> Annie's Naturals salad dressings
> Cardini's salad dressings
> Paul Newman's Own salad dressings
> Nasoya Nayonaise (Tofu salad dressing)
> Nasoya Vegi dressings
> Spectrum canola mayonnaise
> Spectrum Lite canola mayonnaise
> Spectrum vegetable oils (olive oil, canola, etc.)
> Hain mayonnaise
> Barlean's Fresh Express flax oil

Condiments

When you pay close attention to the labels on the condiments, you'll be amazed at how many condiments are packed
with corn syrup, dextrin, monosodium glutamate (MSG), and
sugar in many forms.   It's almost impossible to find a
spaghetti sauce without high-fructose corn syrup and cotton-
seed oil! In your grocery store, Sutter Home and Classico are
two companies who make tomato sauces without sugar or
hydrogenated oils.

At the local health food store, look for the brand Enrico's
or any of the other wonderful home-style cooked tomato
sauces. Many of my clients prefer Bragg's Amino Acids in
place of salt or soy sauce. Your health food store also has
sugar-free condiments.

> Bernard Jensen's vegetable broth and seasoning
> Bragg's Liquid aminos
> Westbrae or Tree of Life Dijon mustard

Westbrae Tamari soy sauce (low sodium)
Eden soy sauce
Sutter Home tomato sauce
Classico tomato sauces (read labels; some varieties contain sugar)
Enrico's spaghetti sauces and condiments
Tree of Life spaghetti sauce
Muir Glen spaghetti sauce
Bragg's Apple cider vinegar, raw, unpasteurized
Brown Rice vinegar (Spectrum Foods)
San-J Wheat-Free tamari
Beeritos salsa
Hain barbecue sauce
Hain chili sauce

Jams and Jellies/Nut Butters

After the condiments, we came to the section containing all the jams and jellies. My client and I read labels for almost twenty minutes before we found some jams and jellies without added sugar (high fructose corn syrup) and hydrogenated oils!

The best choices in your grocery store are Smucker's and Polaner's jams. They're sweetened simply with fruits and fruit juices. Below I've listed additional nut butters like those made with almonds, or sesame seeds. Children especially love the taste of natural almond butter. I've also added non-sweetened applesauce to the list since many of the varieties are loaded with sugar. Musselman's was the only one we could find in the grocery store that did not have added sugar. Your health food store will have more choices.

Smucker's Natural peanut butter
Smucker's simply fruit
Arrowhead Mills almond butter, peanut butter, cashew butter, sesame tahini
Apple butter (unsweetened)
Musselman's natural applesauce

Polaner's jams
Maranatha nut butters (almond, cashew, macadamia
   nut, sunflower)

Breads

Another overwhelming place is the bread aisle. My client and I looked at loaf after loaf before we found natural, whole-grain breads. Two names to look for in your grocery stores are Orowheat and Earth Grains. Most health food stores carry Ezekiel Bread, which is a wonderful whole grain-bread, based on a Bible recipe (Ezekiel 4:9). Look for sprouted, seven- or ten-grain breads. Locally, your grocery store might carry variations like nine- or eleven-grain breads. If they're really made with whole-grains, they're great. But don't eat too many servings of bread. Here are some selections to look for.

   Orowheat Honey whole wheat, oat nut, dark rye and
      seven grain, whole wheat
   Serenity Farms unyeasted and yeasted flat breads
   Shiloh Farms
   Earth Grains whole-wheat bread
   Wheat 'N Honey pocket bread
✳ Ezekiel Bread
   Garden of Eatin' breads
   Garden of Eatin' whole-wheat tortillas
   Garden of Eatin' whole-grain pita bread
   Nature's Garden breads
   Nine-grain or sprouted bagels
   Bran muffins
   Whole-grain hamburger buns
   Rye crisp crackers
   Ak-Mak whole-wheat crackers
   Manna sprouted bread

Cereals and Whole Grains

Judging from labels on common breakfast cereals, most kids in America are eating fat and sugar for breakfast! It's hard to find a cereal which contains lower than 3 or 4 grams of sugar per serving. Some are as high as 13 grams (even in the health food store)! In your grocery store, those listed below are the best. Avoid obvious high-fat cereals which includes granola—a high-fat and high-sugar cereal! Not a good choice for weight loss. Brands to look for in the health food stores are Arrowhead Mills, Barbara's, Health Valley, Lundberg and New Morning. Whole-grain waffles (Nutrigrain) are the best bet for waffles, but only occasionally because they are highly processed and can cause weight gain.

Besides oatmeal, brown rice is another cereal grain, much preferred over white rice, which has been refined. Brown rice comes in several varieties. Other options are quinoa, millet, or spelt. These are extremely nutritious grains; however, you may have to get used to their unusual flavors.

Barbara's shredded spoonfuls
Fiber One
Kashi (not puffed)
Kashi Good Friends (8 grams fiber per 3/4 cup)
Health Valley muesli
Roman Meal cream of rye
Roman Meal old fashioned oats
All Bran cereal
Grape Nuts
Barbara's Breakfast O's
Shredded Wheat
Slow Cooking oatmeal
Arrowhead Mills bran or corn flakes
Health Valley oat bran flakes
New Morning honey almond oatios
Uncle Sam's cereal (with flax)
Uncle Ben's brown rice
Arrowhead Mills short and long-grain brown rice

Arrowhead Mills wild rice (quick)
Arrowhead Mills quinoa (whole grain)
Arrowhead Mills millet (whole grain)
Arrowhead Mills spelt flakes

Pasta

Most pastas are made with—you guessed it—refined white flour so they can make you fat. What are better options? First, look for "colored" pasta, which are at least made with spinach, beets or other vegetables. Hodgson Mills is a common grocery store brand. Pritikin, Deboles and Tree of Life makes delicious whole-wheat spaghetti and linguini. Wouldn't it be great if Italian restaurants used natural whole-grain pasta? Your health food store carries many varieties.

Cleopatra's Kamut pasta
Pritikin whole wheat linguini
Pritikin whole wheat spaghetti
Debole's pasta (many varieties, including whole wheat)
Tree of Life pasta (not whole grain)
Fantastic pasta and beans
Vita Spelt pasta
Bionaturea Organic pasta, whole wheat

Proteins

If you can get "organically grown" sources of meat, dairy or fish, then purchase those. Otherwise, select the leanest you can find and use red meat (preferably organically grown) in moderation.

I omit shellfish (lobster, crab, shrimp and oysters) because they are scavengers, and they are higher in saturated fat. Healthy, clean fish have fins and scales which are cleaning filters. Scavengers eat anything and everything, even toxic waste. This waste is stored in their bodies.

"Free range" means the chickens were allowed to roam freely—not penned up. If they aren't exercising, they get fat, just like us! The leaner the meat, the better for you.

Shelton is a manufacturer of organic chickens and turkeys. Shelton also makes wonderful canned Chicken Chili and Turkey Chili, found in your health food store. Other canned meat includes tuna fish packed in water, plus canned chicken and salmon.

Organically-grown eggs and dairy are great. Eggland's best eggs are also good too. Eat natural cheeses moderately.

Vegetarian proteins include beans, grains, and soy foods. Read labels on canned beans because many of them contain sugar and lard! Look for just beans, water and salt. Heinz and Progresso are good grocery store brands. Arrowhead Mills, Health Valley, Hain, Westbrae, and Shelton are manu-facturers of beans that you can find in the health food store.

Soy foods are becoming popular for their health benefits. Soy milk is wonderful, but look one low in sugar. Tempeh is made from beans and rice, and can be used in recipes in place of hamburger or bacon (See Lightlife product Fakin' Bacon). Tofu is like a cheese and it has different styles. Firm tofu is good for a stir-fry, puddings and dips; and soft or silken tofu makes better protein drinks. Boca burgers are soy burgers that are flavored. Many of my clients really like them served on a whole-wheat bun with mustard.

Proteins

Animal Sources:	Vegetarian Sources
Meat	**Beans** (Westbrae, Eden, Bearito,
Ground turkey breast	Heinz, Progresso)
Buffalo meat	Aduki
Chicken breast (skinless)	Black beans
Cornish hen	Black eyed peas

Ground chicken or turkey
Canned chicken or white
Venison
Fish
Bass
Bluefish
Catfish
Cod
Flounder
Haddock
Halibut
Mackerel
Mahimahi
Ocean Perch
Orange Roughy
Red Snapper
Salmon
Sardines
Snapper
Trout
Tuna
Whitefish
Tuna packed in water
Canned salmon in water
Canned sardines in water

Fava
Garbanzo
Great Northern
Kidney
Lentils
Lima
Mung
Navy
Pinto
Peas, green
Red beans
Split peas

Soybean Products
Tofu
Tempeh
Baked, flavored tofu
Ready-ground tofu
Tofu burgers
Boca Burgers
Soy Dream
Pacific soy milk
Soy Moo (Health Valley)
Eden soy milk
Westbrae soy milk
Soylecious (Frozen Dessert)
Yves Veggie tofu wieners
Yves Veggie burgers
Lightlife smart dogs
Lightlife fakin' bacon
Lightlife smart ground
Lightlife smart deli
Lightlife meatless lightburgers

Healthy Fats and Oils

You probably know it's hard to find non-hydrogenated spreads. A great substitute for margarine is Spectrum Spread which is made from canola oil. Also, make your own "better butter" by mixing together equal parts of olive oil and half butter. Use cold-pressed vegetable oils like olive oil and canola oil. You can find various types of olive oil at your grocery store. However, I recommend that you buy other oils, like canola oil or safflower at a health food store, since most grocery stores carry refined oils.

Vegetable sprays like Tyson's or Pam's pump spray are good. Your health food store has healthier alternatives.

Raw butter
Spectrum Spread
Bionaturea olive oil
Spectrum cold-pressed natural oils
Spectrum cold-pressed extra virgin olive oil
Barlean's flaxseed oil
Spectrum cold-pressed sunflower, canola and sesame oil
Avocado
Nature's Cuisine all-natural olive oil spray
Almonds, raw
Arrowhead mills sunflower seeds
Arrowhead mills sesame seeds
Arrowhead mills flaxseeds
Pecans, raw
Pistachio nuts, raw
Walnuts, raw
Cashews, raw
Pumpkin seeds, raw

Dairy

You'll notice I'm not a "got milk" advocate. In working with people over these years, we've seen that dairy is best eaten "pre-digested," as in yogurt, cottage, buttermilk and kefir. You may not be familiar with kefir, but it's a delicious cultured food most often found like a drinkable milk with fruit added.

Eliminate obvious "processed" cheeses that are individually wrapped. Your best bets are natural cheeses, without added colorings. Use cheese very moderately—just one or two tablespoons in a topping to replace that cup of cheese.

Organic Valley milk
Alta Dena milk
Alta Dena buttermilk
Alta Dena kefir
Alta Dena Nonfat, plain yogurt (sweetened with juices)
Chino Valley (free range)
Alta Dena Low fat or raw cottage cheese
Tree of Life Low fat or raw cottage cheese
Eggs (organic, or Eggland's Best)
Butter
Acidophilus milk
Buttermilk, low fat
Mozzarella, part skim
Parmesan cheese
Natural Farmer's cheese
Romano cheese
Feta cheese

Miscellaneous for Cooking

Your family will appreciate a few snacks, so why not stock up on some healthier ingredients for your special baking? Substituting whole-grain pastry flour cup-for-cup for white flour works in most recipes. Your natural foods store has a variety of cookbooks to help you.

Body Ecology stevia powder
Stevita Stevia powder
Sucanat
Mori-Nu Tofu Mates (lemon, vanilla and chocolate
   pudding mixes)
Wonderslim 100% caffeine-free cocoa
Rumford's Non-aluminum baking powder
Ener-G egg replacer
Wonderslim Egg and fat replacer
Sucanat Organic (natural, raw) sugar
Maple Syrup (pure)
Arrowhead Mills Pancake mixes, whole grain
Vanilla (pure)
Bob's Red Mill whole-wheat flour
Bob's Red Mill whole-wheat pastry flour
Arrowhead Mills whole-wheat flour
Arrowhead Mills whole-wheat pastry flour
Powdered skim milk
Real salt
DeSauza's Solar sea salt
Tree of Life maple syrup
Shady Maple Farms maple syrup

Fast Food Health Food

One of the most common complaints I receive from my clients is "How can I make healthy meals that my family likes, like macaroni and cheese?" Find healthier ingredients. For example, Sheila Schmidt, a friend and client makes homemade lasagna using a healthy spaghetti sauce, whole-wheat lasagna noodles and healthy cheeses. You'll find healthier packaged and frozen versions of these foods at your health food store. Amy's is a common brand. Look for:

Taste Adventure's dry soups, chilis, and instant beans
Whole-grain burritos
Amy's pizza

Amy's lasagna
American Puree entrees
Cedarland entrees
Amy's entrees
Lundberg Farms packaged meals
Fantastic packaged meals and meals in a cup
Health Valley soups, packaged meals and meals in a cup
Fantastic Foods rice and beans
Fantastic Foods taboolie
Fantastic Foods burger mix
Arrowhead Mills quick brown rice
Cascadian Farms Frozen Meals: Morrocan,
    Mediterranean, Cajun, Oriental
Chow mein noodles
Water chestnuts
Bamboo shoots
Canned pasta sauces
Canned tomatoes and tomato sauce
Imagine Foods Aseptic pack soups and sauces
Pacific Organic Aseptic pack sauces and broths (dairy and non-dairy)

Healthy Beverages

Going down the beverage aisle in the grocery store is another shocker. The majority of beverages were packed with sugar. Many so-called fruit juices are not real fruit juice, but rather fruit drinks. Look for 100% orange juice with no sugar added. Gatorade, for example, contains water sweetened with sugar and chemicals. Better choices include:

Pure water
Teecino herbal coffee
Cafix, Pero, or Postum
Chinese green tea
Herbal teas: (Try a Celestial Seasonings Sampler pack)
    Chamomile
    Red Zinger
    Mint tea

Rosehips
Sleepy Time
Wild Berry
Peppermint
Raja's cup (Antioxidant tea)
Organic coffee (drink sparingly)
Alta Dena Yogurt Drinkables (yogurt drink)
Perrier water
Campbell's tomato juice
Lemon water
Gerolsteiner mineral water
Freshly squeezed fruit and vegetable juices
R. W. Knudsen juices
Mountain Sun Juices
Eden Soy Milk
Westbrae Soy Milk
Soy Dream
Soy Moo
Naturally Almond (almond drink)
Soy Dream

Healthy Snack Foods

Sheila also told me her children were delighted when they tasted the "healthy" snacks available. Here are some suggestions for your next "snack attack!" Health Valley makes many types of low-fat, healthy snacks, cereal bars, granola bars, and so on.

Wasa Bread crackers
Kavli All Natural whole-grain crispbread
Garden of Eatin' blue chip corn chips
Garden of Eatin' bean chips
Health Valley nonfat granola bars
Health Valley fat-free cookies
Pride O' the Farm whole-wheat fig bars
Heaven Scent low-fat cookies
Frozen fruit bars

Non-fat frozen yogurt (eat sparingly)
Westbrae cookies
Rye Crisp
Tree of Life saltines
Bearitos no-fat snacks
Guitless Gourmet baked chips
Barbara's fat-free fig bars
Mori-Nu Tofu Mates

Chapter Three

Finding Flavor
With Herbs and Spices

Why use herbs? Not only do they help to replace salt and sugar, but they also offer wonderful flavor with no fat or calories which help create variety for your menus. I began cooking with herbs and spices because my early cooking classes were for people who were watching the amount of fat and salt they ate. I soon discovered flavor can come from vegetables like garlic or ginger, vinegars, herbs, spices, lemon juice, and sauces such as Tamari soy sauce. Most cultures have characteristic herbs, like chilies from Mexico or garlic from Italy.

Low-salt salsas either homemade or bottled enhance any Mexican style dish. Brown rice vinegar, apple cider vinegar or the flavored vinegars like raspberry, make delicious dressings and salsas. Vegetable, bean and pasta purees can add flavor without extra fat. And finally, fruit juices and purees enhance flavor in both cooking and baking. Another delicious option is stone ground or Dijon mustard which also contains some salt.

Herbs and Spices

Traditional cultures of Europe and the Far East have used herbs and spices which were valued not only for cooking, but also for their medicinal properties. According to Eastern Indian medicine, each spice contains certain properties that have specific medicinal effects. Indian cooks, for example, prepare meals around predominantly starchy foods like rice, chapati and legumes with the addition of spices and herbs such as garlic and ginger to balance the food and make it more digestible.

Americans are used to two primary flavors, salt and sugar, but there are other flavors used in traditional cooking that are just as satisfying once you are exposed to them. In this cookbook, I try to use spices from each of the taste groups:

Sweet: Honey, dates, licorice, wheat, milk, rice, raisins, and bananas. Example: rice pudding with raisins.

Salty: Sea salt, Tamari, miso, kelp, and seaweeds. Example: salted snacks.

Sour: Vinegar, lemons, green grapes, cheese, tamarind and yogurt. Example: sweet and sour dishes

Bitter: Spinach, kale, green leafy vegetables, rhubarb, and dandelion root. Example: classic spinach salad or spinach tofu quiche.

Spicy or Pungent: Chili peppers, onions, garlic, ginger, jalapeno, cumin, cayenne and black pepper. Example: Mexican salsas with chili peppers.

Astringent: Pomegranate, turmeric, beans and legumes. Example: Bean soup.

Herbs are the plant or leaves of a plant, such as chives, mint or thyme. They draw out the natural flavor of the food they are combined with. Spices, on the other hand, create a new flavor. Spices generally come from the bark, roots, fruit or berries of shrubs or trees. A plain dish can be transformed into a gourmet delicacy with the addition of some freshly-ground spices.

It's generally better to use too little than too much when you first start adding herbs to your cooking. Chili and cayenne are potent and when overused, are difficult to tone down! Follow directions carefully if there is a recommended amount. Generally, to replace one tablespoon of fresh herbs, use 1 teaspoon of dried or 1/2 teaspoon of ground herbs.

Storing herbs is important. Fresh herbs are best, but you can also purchase dried herbs from your natural foods store. Store them in small bottles with tight-fitting lids in a cool, dry place—not on top of the stove, or on the window sill.

Since most vegetarian food themes are inspired by various cultures, I've listed several blends that are good for certain types of foods. For example, I've made "Spanish Brown Rice" (page 192) by pulling from the Mexican blends, and "Curried Chicken and Vegetables" (page 170) using the Indian spices. Always start with 1/2-1/4 teaspoon of herbs and increase slowly. Many stores carry seasonings already blended, several of which are salt-free. An herb glossary is included in Appendix E, on page 246. Here are some combinations:

*Italian: Basil, bay, oregano, marjoram, garlic, parsley, onion, rosemary, thyme, and sage.

Uses: Tomato sauces, pizza sauce, and salad dressings.

*East Indian: Cinnamon, nutmeg, cloves, mace, cardamom, ginger root, turmeric, cumin, coriander, black pepper, fenugreek, mustard seed, and tarragon. These also make a blend of curry powders.

Uses: Beans, rice, vegetables, lentils, dips, sauces and dressings.

*Japanese/Chinese: Ginger root, celery seed, garlic, pepper, mustard, sesame seeds, lemon peel, onion, vinegar, and plum sauce.

Uses: Sweet-and-sour-dishes made from vinegar and honey-type base are nice with vegetables, beans, salads and rice. Gingered flavoring goes well with carrots, vegetable dishes and tempeh.

*Mexican: Paprika, cayenne, cumin, chili, garlic, onion, and red pepper.

Uses: Almost all grain and bean dishes; potatoes, dressings and soups.

*French: Chervil, parsley, marjoram, savory, thyme, fennel, and Dijon mustard.

Uses: Nice in salads, soups and breads. Dijon makes a great flavoring in dressings, lentils, mustard sauce, coleslaw, and tempeh dishes.

*European: Anise, bay, caraway, fenugreek, oregano, parsley, rosemary, poppy seed, savory, thyme, peppermint, celery seed, dill, fennel, and horseradish.

Uses: Breads, vegetable dishes and soups. Dill goes well with soups, breads, dips and dressings.

*Cajun spices: Cayenne, parsley, paprika, garlic, thyme and basil.

Uses: Vegetables and stew.

Occasionally, I'll have some nice vegetables or fruits on hand and look for a new way to prepare them. Here are some nice combinations for various food preparation. Generally, use ¼-½ teaspoon of single herbs and combine one or two herbs to start, gradually adding more herbs to taste.

For sweet vegetables, fruits or desserts: Allspice, cinnamon, cloves, nutmeg, mace, ginger, coriander, curry, orange peel, lemon peel, and vanilla.

For cooking vegetable dishes, salads, and sauces: Onion and garlic; dill and caraway; marjoram and thyme; basil, bay and onion; basil, sage and oregano; garlic, sage, rosemary and thyme.

For salad dressings: Basil, oregano, parsley, rosemary and thyme; garlic and basil; mint, lemon, dill, oregano and parsley, garlic and onion; onion, bay, fennel, rosemary, sage, savory and marjoram.

For cooking beans: Ginger root; kombu seaweed; cumin; fenugreek; savory; sage; onions; garlic; basil; bay leaf. Combinations: cumin and coriander; fenugreek, fennel and dill; chili powder, cayenne and cumin; dill, bay and celery; onion, garlic, cumin and chili powder; cumin, garlic, coriander, and chili powder.

For cooking sweet curries or rice: Ginger, nutmeg, cumin, cardamom, cinnamon, turmeric, cayenne, cloves.

For Indian curries: Turmeric, cumin, coriander, cinnamon, ginger, garlic; or cumin, coriander and turmeric.

PART THREE

Life Design
Meal Planning

Chapter Four

Why Eat Your Veggies?

When were you taught to eat foods that burn fat? I ate what Mom taught me to eat, and she ate what her Mom taught her to eat. Well, who taught their Moms? And what about our schools? Most schools now have vending machines for soda and junk food. Most TV commercials, magazines and books contradict each other so much that everyone is confused about what to eat!

You have to go out of your way to know what to eat. If you only followed the media, print advertising and commercials, you might try to live on processed cereals for breakfast, fast food for lunch, and some type of macaroni or pasta dish for supper like I did many years ago! For many years, we have followed inaccurate guidance about the foods we have eaten. We didn't have any scientific reason for the choices we made. We just ate what we liked because it tasted good.

But we can make choices based on solid scientific research on how your body really works. Have you ever heard of anyone having a soda deficiency or chocolate ice cream deficiency? No, but we can have a folic acid deficiency from not eating leafy green vegetables. We can have a vitamin C deficiency from not eating any oranges, strawberries, tomatoes or red peppers. We can have a fiber deficiency from not eating any apples, whole grains or oatmeal.

Almost daily, my clients ask me how they can eat to get the right nutrition. I suggest they eat lots of whole foods, including a variety of fresh fruits and vegetables.

I tell them to make wise selections based on what your body needs, not based on what tastes good or looks the best. Compare for example, the nutrition in a cup of coffee and a bagel versus a protein shake with some type of milk with fruit. There are no vitamins or minerals in coffee, and most bagels are made of white flour, which means there is little if any nutrition there. The protein shake contains protein, calcium from the milk, and vital vitamins and minerals in the fruit.

How about lunch? The average fast-food burger and fries meal with a soda contains some protein, but is dangerously lacking in cancer-preventing fruits and vegetables. Soda can make you gain weight, and worse yet, the phosphoric acid levels can contribute to bone loss. Compare that lunch to a whole-grain pita, wrap, or sandwich with lean beef or chicken, leaf lettuce, tomatoes, and avocado with a piece of fruit for dessert. This meal contains lots of protein, vitamins C, B, E, many minerals, and essential fat.

Most people eat about 21 meals every week. You can fill a larger amount of the RDAs or required daily allowances by eating healthy balanced meals on a regular basis.

Where Are Your Vegies?

Most of us eat salads for lunch only on occasion. We'll have a side order of cabbage slaw with a burger or a carrot salad at the deli. But salads are wonderful. The best part is they can boost your metabolism. Vegetables have the fewest calories and the most nutrients. Clinical research shows that many vegetables popular in the Mediterranean Region have numerous health benefits such as:

•Natural weight loss

•Increased energy

•Reduced cravings

•Stronger immune system

•Lowered risk of cancer and heart disease

•Improved digestion and elimination

•Healthy weight loss

•Reduced sugar cravings

•Delayed aging process

Generally speaking certain vegetables have phytochemicals which can increase our immunity against heart disease, and help lower cholesterol. They have been proven to reduce the incidence of breast, prostate and colon cancers. Broccoli, cauliflower and cabbage, for example, have phytochemical compounds that boost the production of anti-cancer enzymes within hours after they are eaten.

Both vegetables and fruits with the deepest colors, like red, orange and green yield the highest antioxidant protection. Lutein, found in kale and broccoli, can protect the macula of the eye and a deficiency of lutein has been linked with macular degeneration.

Lycopene is a carotenoid like beta carotene which is also a powerful antioxidant against cancers and is found in foods like tomatoes, red grapefruit, red peppers and watermelon.

Greens are high in chlorophyll. They are also high in iron, magnesium, calcium, manganese, vitamin C, potassium, vitamin A and some of the essential fatty acids. The darker the color, the higher the level of nutrients.

Here is a selection of health-promoting foods you can choose from in planning your daily meals.

Apples: Apples can lower blood cholesterol, blood pressure and the risk for cancer. High in soluble fiber, they help prevent sharp mood swings or stabilize blood-sugar levels; they contain a natural appetite suppressant, and are extremely high in potassium.

Apricots: Apricots are a super source of beta carotene and vitamin C, which may help protect against lung cancer; they are also high in potassium.

Asparagus: Asparagus is high in chlorophyll and vitamin A, and is also helpful for the kidneys.

Avocados: Avocados are good for lowering cholesterol; they benefit circulation and are known for being a rich source of glutathione, a powerful antioxidant. Avocados are high in potassium.

Bananas: Bananas soothe the stomach, prevent and heal ulcers, and help lower cholesterol because of their high amounts of soluble fiber. Bananas help guard against a potassium deficiency. They are rich in B6 which is essential for maintaining a strong immune system.

Barley: Barley is high in a special fiber that can lower the risk of heart disease by lowering LDL, the bad cholesterol. Barley contains some cancer-inhibiting elements. Barley is used mostly in soups.

Beans, whole: Beans are high in protein, fiber, and complex carbohydrates for energy. They help reduce LDL cholesterol and increase HDL cholesterol. Their insoluble fiber helps prevent colon cancer and regulate blood-sugar levels.

Bell pepper, red and green: Rich in vitamin C, peppers help fight off colds, asthma, bronchitis, atherosclerosis and cancer.

Berries: Berries contain an antiviral agent and are helpful for urinary tract infections, especially cranberries and blueberries. Berries are high in insoluble fiber and potassium which helps control blood pressure.

Beets: Beets are high in calcium and potassium. Beets are nourishing to the liver and gallbladder, and are helpful for digestive problems.

Broccoli: Broccoli is full of fiber, beta carotene and vitamin C. It's also high in bone-building calcium and boron. Broccoli is one of the best anti-cancer vegetables, high in sulforaphane, a powerful antioxidant.

Brown rice: Brown rice contains a high amount of B vitamins and is soothing to the nervous system and stomach, healing to the lungs and colon and provides bran for efficient waste elimination.

Brussels Sprouts: Brussels sprouts are high in vitamin C, low in sodium, high in potassium and fiber. They are known to inhibit cancer, especially cancer of the colon and stomach.

Buckwheat: Buckwheat is a high protein seed which contains several amino acids. It's high in complex carbohydrates and B vitamins. Buckwheat can help lower blood cholesterol and help balance blood sugars.

Cabbage: Cabbage is low in calories, high in fiber, high in vitamin C, and is a cancer-preventing food. Cabbage is said to prevent ulcers and kill bacteria and viruses. The juice stimulates the immune system, and cabbage assists in detoxing the liver.

Carob: Carob is a low-sugar, low-sodium, high-potassium and high-fiber food, often used as a replacement for chocolate in candy.

Carrots: Carrots have been shown to cut the risk of lung cancer, and reduce the blood fats that cause heart attacks and strokes. Carrots are an excellent source of beta carotene, a powerful antioxidant, which is immune boosting and infection fighting. Carrots also help reduce the odds of degenerative eye diseases and are good for healthy skin and teeth. Carrot juice is used in the treatment of severe disease like cancer.

Cauliflower: Cauliflower is also low in calories, fat and sodium, and high in vitamin C, potassium and is a good source of fiber. Cauliflower helps reduce the risk of cancer, particularly colon, stomach and breast cancer.

Cantaloupe: Cantaloupes are high in beta carotene, vitamin C, fiber and B6. Cantaloupes may protect against oral and stomach cancer.

Cherries: Cherries are high in potassium and help prevent tooth decay.

Cranberries: Cranberries contains strong antibiotic properties and are known to help fight bladder infections (real unsweetened cranberry juice).

Celery: Celery helps lower blood pressure and is good for the heart. Celery also contains anti-cancer compounds and has a calming effect on the nervous system. Celery is good for water retention, weight-loss and cancer.

Chick peas (garbanzo beans): Chick peas are packed with protein and fiber and help maintain normal blood-sugar levels.

Corn: Corn is the staple food of the Tarahumara Indians of Mexico who have almost no heart disease. Corn is a good source of iron, zinc and potassium and is low in sodium.

Cucumbers: Cucumbers aid digestion, cleanse the bowels, and are helpful for breaking up cholesterol deposits. Cucumbers help to promote healthy skin.

Eggs: An excellent source of protein, the yolks are especially nutrient dense. They contain lecithin and choline, important nutrients for decreasing plaque formation.

Eggplant: Eggplants contain a substance that inhibits the rise of blood cholesterol.

Figs: Figs help prevent cancer and are anti-ulcer and anti-bacterial foods. They also reduce high-blood pressure. Figs are an excellent source of plant fiber for stabilizing blood-sugar levels.

Fish: Certain Omega 3 fish help lower blood cholestero-levels, blood pressure and high triglycerides and prevent cancer and arthritis. Omega 3 oils are found in cold-water fish such as mackerel, salmon, and tuna.

Flaxseed: One of the richest sources of Omega 3 fatty acids, flax is being used to help a variety of conditions including acne, allergies, arthritis, breast pain, diabetes, heart disease, learning disorders, menopause, obesity and stroke. Dr. Johanna Budwig considers flaxseed one of the best cancer-preventive foods available.

Garlic: Garlic contains substances that help lower blood pressure, reduce cholesterol, and hinder the formation of blood clots. Garlic boosts the immune system and acts as a natural antibiotic.

Ginger: Ginger can treat nausea, stomach aches, and congestion. A natural diet aid, ginger boosts the rate the body burns calories and is a natural antioxidant.

Greens: Greens are high in vitamin A, high in fiber, low in calories, low in fat, and high in minerals.

Grapes: Grapes are a good source of boron, and help ward off osteo-porosis. Red grapes help prevent artery damage and heart attacks, and may lower blood pressure.

Grapefruit: Grapefruits can lower blood cholesterol and can reduce blood fats (triglycerides).

Grains, whole: Whole grains are rich in complex carbohydrates and are rich in fiber which can help reduce the risk of cancer.

Horseradish: Horseradish is said to help asthma, bronchitis and lung disorders.

Kale: Another member of the cruciferous family kale is high in anti-cancer chemicals. Kale is rich in beta carotene and vitamin C which reduces the harmful affects of LDL. Kale is high in calcium which is easily assimilated.

Kiwifruit: Kiwifruit is packed with nutrients, especially vitamin C, fiber and antioxidants.

Leeks: A long onion which looks like a large green onion in the onion family. It's a blood purifier and aid for the liver.

Lemon: Lemons regenerate the liver, strengthen the stomach acids and salivary enzymes, and help the pancreas, thyroid and adrenal glands.

Lentils: Lentils are a high-protein, high-fiber food. They are excellent food for diabetics and protect against high cholesterol.

Mango: Mangos help lower blood pressure, and are high in beta carotene and vitamin C.

Melon: Melons contain the antioxidant beta carotene and are high in fiber, potassium and vitamin C.

Millet: Millet is a small gluten-free grain that makes a good substitute for rice. It has a nice light flavor. It's excellent grain for the spleen, pancreas and stomach.

Mushrooms: Mushrooms such as Reishi and Shitake are said to help prevent and treat cancer, viral disease and high-blood cholesterol.

Mustard Greens: Mustard greens act as a decongestant and help break up mucus in air passages. Mustard greens contain high amounts of calcium, iron, vitamin A and niacin.

Nuts: Nuts contain anti-cancer and heart protective properties. They are full of antioxidants and monosaturated fat, which protect arteries from damage.

Oats: Oats are high in soluble fiber and said to help stabilize the blood-sugar level.

Olive oil: Olive oil improves digestion, and helps decrease gallstone formation. Olive oil helps increase the good cholesterol, decrease bad cholesterol, and helps regulate blood-sugar levels.

Onions: Onions thin the blood, help lower cholesterol, help to prevent strokes and boost HDL, the good cholesterol.

Oranges: Oranges are high in vitamin C and folic acid which fight birth defects. Oranges are rich in antioxidants and beta carotene and may ward off asthma, bronchitis and breast cancer.

Papaya: Papayas are high in Vitamin C and A; and are helpful in digestive problems.

Parsley: Parsley helps the kidneys, bladder, prostate and urinary tract disorders.

Peanuts: Peanuts are rich in fiber, E, copper, magnesium, managenese, and B vitamins.

Peaches: High in Vitamin A, peaches are an alkaline fruit with a laxative effect.

Peas: Peas are a good source of cholesterol-lowering soluble fiber. Peas are known to prevent cancer because of carotene and vitamin C.

Pears: Pears are a great source of fiber, and help reduce the risk of developing polyps of the colon.

Pineapple: Pineapples contain bromelain, an anti-inflammatory. Pineapple is said to aid digestion, dissolve blood clots and help prevent osteoporosis.

Potatoes: Potatoes are high in potassium and are said to help prevent high-blood pressure. They contain anti-cancer substances.

Prunes: Prunes have a laxative effect, and provide relief for constipation. Prunes contain lots of fiber, boron and vitamins A and E.

Pumpkin: Pumpkins are high in beta carotene which has been known to help in cancer, heart attacks and cataracts.

Quinoa: Quinoa is an Incan grain which has a light taste and pleasant texture. It's good in salads, pilafs and soups. Quinoa also contains all the amino acids and is a whole protein.

Radishes: Radishes are said to promote digestion, remove mucus, and soothe headaches. Radishes contain vitamins A, B and C.

Raspberries: High in vitamins A and C, raspberries are great cleansers and aid digestion.

Rye: Rye is a grain which has a strong flavor, and few allergenic reactions. It contains the highest amount of lysine of all the grains, and is low in gluten. Rye can be cooked as a cereal or bread.

Salmon: Salmon is rich in Omega 3 fatty acids, and is a great source of essential fat and protein.

Soybeans: A bean which is high in the antioxidant Genistein, a cancer fighting compound, soybeans provide all nine essential amino acids.

Squash: Squash is high in beta carotene, and is said to lower the risk of cancer, particularly lung cancer. Squash helps heal inflammation, relieve pain and soothe the stomach.

Spinach: Spinach is high in vitamin A (beta carotene) for eye health, calcium, B vitamins and vitamin E.

Strawberries: Strawberries contain more vitamin C and fiber than in most fruits and has antiviral and anti-cancer properties.

Sweet potatoes: (Yams). Sweet Potatoes are high in beta carotene and linked to preventing heart disease.

Tomatoes: A good source of vitamin C, tomatoes aid in cleansing the body of toxins, and help lower the risk of cancers.

Wheat: Wheat is a whole-grain full of vitamins, minerals and bran. It's said to raise good cholesterol levels.

Yogurt: Yogurt is high in protein and calcium and it contains certain bacteria which aid digestion, and help correct constipation.

Vinegar, apple cider: ACV has been used for fighting arthritis and germs and bacteria naturally, and regulating calcium metabolism.

Chapter Five

Easy Meal Planning

Now that we've looked at how foods burn fat, how to set up your kitchen, and the health value of specific foods, let's get down to meal planning based on the philosophy I gave you in chapter one. Eating smaller portion sizes will help you eat a variety of food, too.

Daily Servings

A good eating plan would include:

2-3 servings of protein a day

2 fruit servings a day

5 vegetable servings a day

1-3 carbohydrate servings a day

1 tablespoon of flaxseed oil a day

Daily Serving Sizes

Healthy carbohydrates: Serving size: 1 slice whole-grain bread, ½ cup cooked whole-grain cereal, rice or pasta, 1 cup dry cereal, ½ whole-grain bagel or English Muffin, 3-4 whole-grain crackers, 1 tortilla, 1 whole-grain chapati

Healthy meats: Serving size: 3 ounces poultry, fish or lean meat, 1 egg

Healthy milk, yogurt and cheese: Serving size: 1 cup milk or yogurt, ½ ounces of natural cheese, 2 ounces of processed cheese, ½ cup low-fat cottage cheese

Healthy fats: Serving size: 1 tablespoon flaxseed oil, extra virgin olive oil, expeller pressed canola oil, 10 raw nuts including almonds, cashews, walnuts and hazelnuts; ¼ cup seeds such as sesame seeds and sunflower seeds

Healthy vegetables: Serving size: 1 cup raw, leafy vegetables, ½ cup chopped or cooked vegetables, ¾ cup of vegetable juice

Healthy fruits: Serving size: 1 piece of fruit, 4 ounces of juice, ½ cup canned fruit, ¼ cup dried fruit, 1 cup berries

Vegetarian serving size to replace milk and dairy: 1 cup soymilk, ½ cup tofu or tempeh, 1 soy burger, 2 soy hot dogs, 3 ½ tablespoons soy protein powder

Vegetarian serving size to replace meat: ½ cup cooked beans or peas, two tablespoons of peanut butter, ¼ cup (1 ounce) nuts, ¼ cup seeds

Plan Your Weekly Meals

Most people feel overwhelmed when they first start planning meals. Here are some tips:

1. Find a time to plan your meals for the week, for example, an hour on a Saturday or Sunday afternoon.

2. Write out the meals you want to make for the week.

3. Make a shopping list of the foods needed for these recipes. Inventory the foods you have on hand, and go over each recipe, jotting down the type and amount of foods you need.

4. Take the list with you and buy the foods you need for the week.

Sample Meal Plan

Upon Arising: *Lemon Drink (Recipes have an asterisk (*)

Breakfast

1. *Oatmeal or Oat Bran (with small amount of protein like egg or cottage cheese) or

2. *Protein Drink or *Smoothie or

3. *Poached eggs with one slice of whole grain toast and butter.

Herbal tea or water

Lunch

(Choose from a large vegetable salad, animal or vegetable protein and complex carbohydrate)

1. Chicken Caesar Salad with one slice of whole-grain bread.

2. Tuna fish salad on whole-grain bread with lettuce, tomato and cucumber.

3. Vegetable and beef stew with one slice Ezekial 4:9 bread.

Dinner

1. Chili with green salad and three whole-grain crackers.

2. Grilled chicken breast sandwich with lettuce, tomato and cucumber on whole-grain bread.

3. Grilled Salmon, steamed broccoli and carrots, and ½ cup brown rice.

Herbal tea or water

Snacks

½ cup cottage cheese with fruit

½ cup non-fat yogurt with fruit

Protein drink or protein bar
10 raw nuts or seeds
Raw vegetable sticks
2 Wasa bread crackers with 1 slice natural cheese
2 Kavli Crispbread with chicken strips and Dijon mustard
Tuna fish on whole-grain crackers
8-10 almonds
1/4 cup macadamia nuts
8-10 pistacio nuts 4-5 pecans
1/4 cup sunflower seeds
1/4 cup cashews
4-6 pine nuts
1 ounce cashew butter, almond butter or peanut butter on 1 whole grain cracker.

1 ounce string cheese, or Feta cheese, or Swiss cheese, or Mozzarella cheese, or Cheddar cheese with 3-4 whole grain crackers or one piece of fruit.

Vegetarian Alternatives

Here are some vegetarian alternatives for my vegetarian readers.

• Make the protein drink with soy milk or tofu.

• Make the Tofu Dressing or Tofu "Eggless" Salad.

• Cube and sauté tofu in a stir-fry with vegetables.

• Substitute Boca Burger or Lightlife Meatless Burger for Turkey Burgers.

• Have brown rice with grilled tofu and a side salad.

• Have a hearty vegetable bean stew with side salad and whole-grain bread.

•Use black beans, red beans or chili in place of animal
  protein.
•Use Fakin' Bacon or grilled tempeh in place of
  grilled chicken.
•Grate tempeh with a cheese grater, and lightly sauté
  in a small amount of olive oil and use in place of
  hamburger meat. Or grill tempeh on a grill with a
  small amount of olive oil. I've given a vegetarian
  substitute in each of these meals.

Seven Days of Menus

On the following pages, I have given you menus for
seven days. I've included both animal and vegetable
protein suggestions.

**Recipes which are included in this book have an
asterisk (*) next to them.**

Day One (Upon arising: *Lemon Drink)

Breakfast
  *Protein drink or *Smoothie (or fruit if appropriate) or
  *Oatmeal and 1 egg or cottage cheese
    Herbal tea or water

Lunch
  *Grilled Caesar Chicken salad or Caesar Salad with
  Fakin' Bacon strips
  1 slice whole-grain bread
  Herbal tea or water

Dinner
  *Dijon Perch or *Honey Baked Beans
  *Greek Salad
  2 rye crackers
  Herbal tea or water

Day Two (Upon arising: *Lemon Drink)

Breakfast
  *Protein drink or *Smoothie (or fruit if appropriate) or
  *Oatmeal and 1 egg or cottage cheese
    Herbal tea or water

Lunch
  Turkey chili (Shelton's brand from health food store) or
  *Simple Chili
  *Mexican Taco Salad
  *No-Oil Italian Dressing
    1 slice whole-grain bread and butter
    Herbal tea or water

Dinner
  *Lemon Baked Halibut or *Greek Lentils
  *Classic Mixed Green Salad
    Baked potato
    Herbal tea or water

Day Three (Upon arising: *Lemon Drink)

Breakfast
  *Protein drink or *Smoothie (or fruit if appropriate) or
  *Oatmeal and 1 egg or cottage cheese
    Herbal tea or water

Lunch
  Large Vegetable Salad
  *Basic Italian Dressing or *Tofu Dijon dressing
  Baked chicken breast or Lightlife Meatless Burger
  3 small new potatoes
  Herbal tea or water

Dinner
  Steamed vegetables (carrots, broccoli, cauliflower)
  3 ounces fish or chicken (baked or grilled, not fried)
  or grilled tempeh
  1 slice whole-grain bread
  Herbal tea or water

Day Four (Upon arising: *Lemon Drink)

Breakfast
    *Protein Drink or *Smoothie (or fruit if appropriate) or
    *Oatmeal and 1 egg or cottage cheese
      Herbal tea or water

Lunch
    *Grilled Caesar Chicken salad or *Grilled Chicken
      Caesar Salad with Fakin' Bacon strips
      1 slice whole-grain bread
      Herbal tea or water

Dinner
    *Chicken Oriental Stir-fry or stir-fry with tofu
    ½ cup *Basic Brown Rice
    *Classic Mixed Green Salad
      Herbal tea or water

Day Five (Upon arising: *Lemon Drink)

Breakfast
    *Protein Drink or *Smoothie (or fruit if appropriate) or
    *Oatmeal and 1 egg or cottage cheese
      Herbal tea or water

Lunch
    *Herbed Chicken or Boca Burger on a wheat bun
      Healthy Coleslaw
      1 baked yam

Dinner
    *Chicken Cacciatore or *Spicy Black Beans
    *Greek Salad
      1 slice whole-wheat bread
      Herbal tea or water

Day Six (Upon arising: *Lemon Drink)

Breakfast

*Protein Drink or *Smoothie (or fruit if appropriate) or
*Oatmeal and 1 egg or ½ cup cottage cheese
Herbal tea or water

Lunch

*Easy Baked or Grilled Fish or *Simple Chili
*Salad Nicoise
1 slice whole-grain bread

Dinner

Shelton turkey burger (purchase at health food store)
on wheat bun or *Boca Burger on wheat bun
Healthy Coleslaw
Herbal tea or water

Day Seven (Upon arising: *Lemon Drink)

Breakfast

*Protein Drink or *Smoothie (or fruit if appropriate) or
*Oatmeal and 1 egg or ½ cup cottage cheese
Herbal tea or water

Lunch

*Vegetable Chop Suey
*Easy Salmon Bake or grilled tempeh
½ cup *Oriental Wild Rice

Dinner

*Chicken Italian Style with whole-grain pasta or
Spaghetti with Soy Ground Round and whole-grain pasta
*Classic Mixed Green Salad
Herbal tea or water

More on Meal Planning

Everyone has their own style of change. Some people like to take their time and make changes gradually. Other people take the "jump in the water and swim" approach. That was my style. When I first started to learn how to cook naturally more than 20 years ago, I couldn't wait to learn how to cook beans or make healthy desserts and salads. I totally revamped my kitchen in one weekend! Whatever your style, here are some changes to consider:

1. You may want to substitute rather than throw things away. First, substitute whole-wheat or other whole-grain flours, cereals, breads and pasta for the white processed variety of these foods.

2. Stock your kitchen with more fresh and frozen fruits and vegetables, whole-grain-products, lean meat fish and poultry, and non-fat yogurt instead of canned varieties.

3. Switch from hydrogenated fats (like Crisco) and margarine to cold-pressed oils like canola and olive oil and use small amounts of butter.

4. Consider fish or lean protein as a basis for meal planning. Center a meal around whole grains and beans, tofu or tempeh for a change.

5. Rather than using regular table salt, consider using salt substitutes or Real sea salt, which is healthier and tastes better.

6. Replace white sugar with healthier sweeteners. You can learn more about these in Appendix D, on page 242.

7. Develop a sense for what is whole and natural, and think about where your food comes from. For example, peanut butter is made from peanuts that are simply ground up. The commercial version adds sugar and hydrogenates the peanut butter, which makes it more processed and less

healthy. Generally, the less processing the healthier the food, and the better it tastes.

Make your change fun. Involve your whole family in your menu planning and cooking. Don't get rid of snacks—just make them lower in fat and healthier. If you stock your kitchen with healthy staples, you will eat better.

Chapter Six

Tips for Quick Meals

Has this ever happened to you? You go to the refrigerator, open the door, stand there and just hang out there for a minute. Sometimes you mentally calculate what you could eat, eliminating anything that will take too long. It doesn't always leave a lot of options, because you are tired, hungry, and usually want something quick!

One of the problems that people often have is a lack of time to cook. However, even with little time, you can still make quick, healthy meals. Most people are surprised to see how quickly good, wholesome meals can be to put together. Many of the dishes in this cookbook can be made in twenty minutes or less.

Getting fast food isn't necessarily faster, either. By the time you drive through and wait in a line, you could have already made something far healthier and cheaper.

People often ask me, "How do you cook? Do you spend hours in the kitchen?" While there are many recipes in this book that I love and use, my daily cooking is simple. Years ago I started planning my meals around protein and vegetables and have found it to be the simplest, yet healthiest meal planning. Protein can come from either vegetable or animal sources. Animal protein meals could include a chicken breast with a green salad and a side dish of vegetables. Vegetarian protein meals could include a large vegetable salad accompanied by some type of bean dish like Spicy Chili. Here are some meals that I often make. Most of them are so simple, that children can make them.

Quick Meal Suggestions

Cottage Cheese and Fruit

Combine ½ cup cottage cheese with ½ cup mixed fruit of choice. **Optional:** Add pineapple, mango, strawberries, blueberries.

Egg Omelet on Bagel

I like to cook 1 or 2 eggs and place them on a whole-grain sprouted wheat bagel or whole-grain bread. It's easy to make for a quick breakfast.

Tomato Feta Salad

Cut a tomato, add ¼ ounce feta cheese, ¼ of an avocado, and serve with Italian dressing.

Easy Stir-fry

Use ½ package frozen stir-fry vegetables; ½ package pre-cooked chicken strips; mix together and heat until warm. Serve with olive oil and Oriental seasonings. Serve in a wrap or serve cold as a salad.

Quick Tuna and Veggies

Open a can of tuna, combine it with ½ cup chopped fresh or thawed frozen veggies in a bowel and add a dressing or natural mayonnaise.

Cucumber Chicken and Avocado Salad

Combine ½ cucumber, chopped, ½ avocado, and chopped, ½ red pepper, chopped. Add chicken cubed, with mayonnaise. Serve as a salad or wrap filling.

Ultimate Veggie Taco or Wrap

My friend, Michelle likes to make this easy lunch meal. Make a mixture of avocado, garlic and onion powder. Spread on one-half of a whole-wheat tortilla. Place fresh raw green beans, chopped broccoli, cauliflower and tomatoes on top. Fold over and eat.

Easy Wrap Ideas

(You can also use pita pockets or whole-grain breads)

Start with tuna, chicken or turkey salad. Dice one cup of celery, add 1 teaspoon of salt and 1 cup cooked meat. Moisten with mayonnaise and use as a filling.

Optional: Add 3 chopped pickles, 1 chopped boiled egg, or 1 tablespoon Parmesan cheese.

Veggie Wrap

Combine chopped avocado, cucumber, onion, tomato and lettuce with Ranch dressing or mayonnaise. Stuff in a whole-grain tortilla.

Chicken Wrap

Combine Fahita chicken, sliced red pepper, tomatoes, and grated Mozzarella cheese and stuff in a whole-wheat tortilla.

Beef Wrap

Combine chopped lean beef, tomatoes, lettuce with horse-radish and mayonnaise and stuff in a whole-wheat tortilla .

Easy Pasta Primavera

Combine 1 cup cooked, cooled pasta with steamed broccoli, carrots, and red peppers. Serve with olive oil and a small amount of Parmesan cheese.

Easy Oriental Pasta Salad

Combine 1 cup cooked bowtie pasta with stir-fry frozen veggies (thawed) and olive oil/vinegar dressing, spiked with ginger, soy sauce or Tamari and salt.

Easy Italian Pasta Salad

Combine 1 cup cooked pasta, cooled, with fresh or frozen veggies and serve with Italian dressing.

Low-Fat Pita Pizzas

These are easy and quick.

Crust: Whole-wheat pita bread (or you can use whole-grain tortilla (corn or flour) or whole-wheat chapati).

Sauce: Favorite low-fat pizza sauce or tomato sauce.

Cheese: Fat-free Mozzarella cheese.

Toppings: Chose from the following: chopped onion, mushrooms, green peppers, tomatoes, black olives, and red or green peppers.

Slice pita-bread in half and spread each half with vegetables, sauce and cheese. Bake at 300° F. for about 10-15 minutes.

Below are two variations.

Mexican Pita Pizza

Whole-wheat pita bread

Refried beans or black bean dip

Jalapeno peppers

Fat-free cheddar cheese

Nacho chips

Slice pita bread in half and spread each half with bean dip, toppings (onion, black olives and jalapeno peppers), sauce, cheddar cheese and chips. Bake at 300° F. for 10-15 minutes.

Fruit Pita Pizza

Applesauce

Orange marmelade or berry jam

Sliced bananas, strawberries, kiwi fruit or blueberries

Slice pita bread in half and spread with the bread with applesauce/jam mixture. Lay sliced fruit on top in rows. Top with crumb crust:

Topping:

¼ cup quick-cooking oats or wheat germ

¼ cup whole-wheat pastry flour

2 tablespoon Sucanat or brown sugar

¼ cup applesauce or butter

Combine and mix in a saucepan and gently toast until somewhat crumbly. Spoon over Fruit Pizza.

Top with a fat-free whipped cream, Tofu-Whipped Cream, or Stevia Whipped Cream if desired (see recipe index).

Other Tips for Quick Meals

1. Use time-saving appliances such as food processors, blenders and bread machines when preparing meals.

2. Keep salad vegetables in your refrigerator. Today, there are several pre-washed salad mixes ready to eat in your grocery store. Just grab some chicken strips and a dressing for a quick salad.

3. Use frozen vegetables whenever appropriate. Frozen vegetables are still more nutritious than canned and are often picked at the ripest time. Add near the end of cooking to keep valuable nutrients.

4. A quick lunch is possible with the new instant soups now available in many health food stores and grocery stores. Just add boiling water to a small container of dried grains, beans, or vegetables and spices and let steep for five minutes. These are delicious with some nonfried corn chips and a salad or raw vegetables.

5. Make an entree centered around one of the quick-cooking beans. Red lentils only take 25 minutes with no soaking required; green lentils require no soaking and cook in under 30 minutes; green or yellow split peas require no soaking and take 30-45 minutes to cook. Let cooked beans cool before refrigerating or they may become sour.

6. Use canned beans in place of homemade cooked beans whenever appropriate. Rinse the beans first and drain well to get rid of excess salt. I like buying canned beans in the lead-free cans made by some companies. Get a few cans each week and experiment. These make such a great quick meal. Just open the can, drain if necessary, heat and add some spices, salsa or tomato sauce. Serve with a green salad and corn bread or grain salad and you have a great meal.

7. Experiment with low-salt, low-fat ready-to-eat soy protein foods such as Lightlife's Meatless Lightburgers or

Smart Ground, both made from soy. Tofu and tempeh are available in a ready-to-eat, baked and marinated form, too. Recipes using these foods are in this cookbook. You can freeze both tofu and tempeh.

8. Cook ahead on weekends. When you bake beans, or bake chicken, beef or turkey meat, make a double batch and freeze the rest. Lentils make a nice lentil chili or lentil salad. Most whole natural foods freeze well. Use leftover beans for soup, dips, or even burgers and loaves.

9. Make a main dish using quick-cooking grains like corn grits (polenta), couscous, bulgur wheat, buckwheat (kasha) or quinoa, and add some protein and a vegetable.

10. Millet, buckwheat and amaranth are also fairly quick cooking from 20-30 minutes. If you use brown rice, plan from 50-55 minutes for cooking, cool, and freeze the rest.

11. Make a main dish from quick-cooking spinach, artichoke, or wheat pasta. Most pastas cook in 5 to 10 minutes. They are nice as a main dish or salad and can be combined with vegetables, beans and nuts for variety. Add some protein and vegetables.

Today there are many varieties of frozen and packaged healthy meals that are quick cooking and wholesome, usually available in health food stores. See the list of healthier fast food on pages 36 and 37.

Quick and easy seasonings: The reason I don't use commercial mixes is that so many of them are loaded with extra salt, sugar, some hidden fat, MSG, and loads of preservatives and chemicals. However, there are a few mixes out there that make making a healthy dinner much quicker. Try to find mixes that do not contain MSG, or high amounts of salts or preservatives. You can find these in a natural foods store, or a health food section of your grocery store.

Chili seasoning mixes: Mix a can of beans and some water and mix to make chili in under 20 minutes.

Taco seasoning mixes: Just mix with water and add to either ground beef, turkey, chicken or a vegetable protein like tempeh, which I like to use.

Stir-fry mix: If you want to make a stir-fry in minutes, just sauté your vegetables and chicken in a sauce made with a Stir-fry mix, Tamari soy sauce, and rice or wine vinegar.

Fajita mix: Fajitas are such a wonderful, popular dish. Look for a Fajita mix and add oil and lemon juice to marinate the chicken.

Chapter Seven

Getting Slim
While Eating Out

Many of my clients faithfully eat healthy at home but lose direction when they eat out. They think, "I can eat well at home, but in a restaurant? No way!"

But you can eat out and still lose weight. Let's look at general restaurant tips, eating fast food, and what to order at your favorite ethnic restaurant.

GENERAL RESTAURANT TIPS

Take Your Enzymes

Carry a small container of enzymes in your purse or pocket so you will always have them with you in case of digestive upsets. Just recently, my friend's mother had a stomachache after dinner. Her stomachache left immediately after I gave her digestive enzymes.

Order Lemon Water

Order water with lemon wedges on the side, to further aid the digestion process. Rather than use white sugar or those "pink and blue" packets, use the "brown packets"—sugar in the raw. Better still, carry stevia, which is a naturally safe, sweet herb (see pages 84, and 244-245). I use it to sweeten lemon water (see lemon drink recipe) or herbal tea. You can buy packets of stevia at your health food store.

Have it Your Way!

You have a choice! You have a right to ask questions, or order food how you want it. For example, at a Chinese restaurant you can request food without MSG added. At a French restaurant, you can order fish or chicken grilled, not fried. Or, order a salad with dressing on the side and use their dressing sparingly.

Don't Eat It All Because You Can

Skip the all-you-can-eat buffets. You wind up eating all you can eat. It's great that you can serve yourself, but the fat grams and calories add up fast.

The Skinny on Salad Bars

Wonder why we can still gain weight in spite of the popularity of salad bars? I've seen people make a great salad with vegetables like carrots, cucumbers, broccoli, mushrooms, green peas, and tomato—and then dump lots of high-fat salad dressing on top! Here are better suggestions.

- Just have a taste of salad dressing or any salads prepared with mayonnaise (coleslaw, potato salad, or macaroni salad).
- Try garbanzo beans, kidney beans, and turkey or chicken breast.
- Try nonfat yogurt, ask for low-fat salad dressing, or vinegar and olive oil dressing, or bring your own.
- Skip the cheese, fried noodles, olives, and roasted, salted seeds.

Pick a Healthy Breakfast

- Oatmeal or whole-grain dry cereals with skim milk
- Fresh fruit or fruit salads
- Whole-wheat toast or whole-grain English muffins
- Omelets with vegetables
- Low-fat yogurt with fresh fruit and granola

75

•Herbal tea

•Poached eggs with whole-grain toast

Skip the Appetizers

Don't nibble before you eat! Wherever you eat, skip the bread and butter, and chips and dip. Save room for the nutrient-dense foods such as chicken and vegetables.

Don't Eat Too Much

Most restaurant meals are too big. Just because it's sitting on your plate doesn't mean it has to go in your tummy.

Split a dinner with a friend. Or, take some home for tomorrow's lunch.

Don't Drink!

Drinking alcohol puts fat on your liver and your body. All liquid sugar drinks are empty calories that deplete your vitamin and minerals.

Order Smart

Order entrees prepared in a low-fat way: broiled, steamed, poached, roasted, baked, grilled, or stir-fried. Try grilled or roast turkey, broiled fish, steamed vegetables, and lean meats. Order broiled chicken, chicken breast, or turkey sandwiches and leave off the cheese.

- •Try low-fat, whole-grain breads, mustard, lots of vegetables and lean meats.
- •Choose vegetable, tomato-based, or bean soups rather than creamed or cheese soups. Avoid casseroles.
- •Order a main course of vegetable, a side salad, and chicken appetizers.
- •For dessert, try fruit, fruit sorbets, or angel food cake.

Avoid Artery-Clogging Fat

•Here's the fat you want to avoid:

•Fried chicken, deep-fried foods, fried onion rings

•French fries, creamy sauces and dressings

•Pizza, sandwiches made with fatty meats like bologna, pastrami, sausage, and luncheon meat

•Chips and nachos

WHAT ABOUT FAST FOOD?

Ever wonder what to choose when you're in a rush and the only thing you can grab is "fast food?" Here are some tips and better choices:

•Drink water instead of high sugar beverages. If you are ordering fast food, order a small green salad with dressing on the side.

•Grilled or roasted chicken sandwiches are your best choices.

•Stick with plain burgers, baked potatoes, mashed potatoes, or corn on the cob.

•Salad bar items to choose: greens, cottage cheese, vegetables without dressing, beans, and fruits.

•Try roast turkey, roast chicken, and broiled fish.

•Order sub sandwiches on wheat bread, with turkey or chicken and fresh vegetables. Omit the mayonnaise

•Grilled chicken breast sandwiches, best on whole-wheat bun

•Chicken salad with low-fat dressings or oil and vinegar dressing

•Skip the French fries, onion rings and all fried foods.

•Avoid cheeseburgers and fried chicken.

•Also avoid pizzas, cheese sauces, creamy salad dressings, gravies, and coleslaw.

SPECIALTY RESTAURANTS

American:

- Grilled, steamed or baked lean meats (such as chicken or fish)
- Salads with lean meats, all vegetables
- Use salad dressing on the side, and dip with your fork before each bite. Or ask for lemon juice, vinegar and seasonings.
- Whole-grain breads
- Non-creamy soups
- Whole-bean soups
- Baked potatoes, or better yet, baked yams

Skip:

- French fries
- Gravies and sauces
- Fried chicken
- Potato skins
- Fatty toppings

Mexican

- Spanish rice, rice and bean dishes, gazpacho, or black-bean soup Taco salad, vegetable burrito, refried beans (without lard), Chicken Fajitas or chicken tacos
- Tostadas, burritos or enchiladas made with beans or chicken
- Rice, black beans, salsa, and steamed corn tortillas
- Guacamole or sliced avocado
- Chicken soft tacos with little cheese
- Order extra lettuce and tomato on the side for nutritional value without fat

Skip:

- Flour tortilas (ask for whole-grain tortillas if available)
- Burritos, tostadas, tacos, and enchiladas made with beef, cheese and sausage
- Nachos, con queso, fried tortilla chips, refried beans and corn tamales (both made with lard)
- Hold the sour cream

Italian

- Order a vegetable salad or plain pasta and broiled fish or chicken
- Try pasta with red sauce, marinara sauce, or tomato-based sauces
- Order clear white sauces, not creamy white sauces
- Order lean meats
- Try pasta primavera, minestrone soup, grilled chicken cacciatore, and chicken or veal picatta
- Italian ice is a fat-free dessert, but high in sugar, so only order a small portion if you can handle it

Skip:

- Pesto and cream sauces, and avoid deep-fried dishes, sausages, and salami
- Cheesecake is high calorie and high fat
- Avoid cheese-filled pasta, sausage dishes, cream and butter sauces, beef ravioli and lasagna

Chinese

- Oriental food is not necessarily low fat! Ordering the wrong types of foods can cause you to eat as much fat as Mexican food. I suggest that you go for lower-salt foods. A plus would be real buckwheat (soba) noodles
- If available, order brown rice rather than white rice
- Ask for steamed rather than fried rice
- Order steamed, stir fried, or boiled chicken and fish dishes that include vegetables and rice
- Order clear soups, bean curd, and vegetable dishes
- Most soups are okay unless you know they are made with oil

Skip:

Ask ahead and avoid foods made with monosodium glutamate (MSG) MSG is an additive that makes some people nauseous. It has been known to adversely affect the nervous system
- Avoid deep-fried egg rolls, fried noodles, and deep-fried dishes such as fried dumplings and fried wontons

French

- Try steamed or grilled fish or chicken breast or broiled lean meat
- Order dishes prepared with wine sauces rather than butter or cream sauces
- Choose seafood, poached fish, chicken in wine sauce, and steamed vegetables
- Choose fresh fruits, and cheese, and sorbet for dessert

Skip:

- Avoid au gratin dishes made with cheese, cream sauces, butter sauces, blue cheese, or bernaise sauce (all made with eggs, butter, or cheese)
- Avoid rich pastries

Japanese

- Order grilled fish or chicken teriyaki, sukiyaki, stir-fried vegetables and broth-based soups
- Order noodle soups and broth, bean sprouts and tofu
- Also try miso or bean soups, udon noodles, steamed rice and rice noodles

Skip:

- Avoid fried foods such as tempuras, fried chicken and fried pork
- Avoid raw fish

Greek

- Order shish kabob, grilled fish, grilled chicken,
- Yogurt and cucumber dishes, rice pilaf and salads (have a few olives and small amount of feta cheese)
- Also try legumes bean soups or lentil soup, eggplants, lentil soup, and grape leaves

Skip:

- Deep fried dishes, creamy dishes, anchovies and baklava

PART FOUR

Easy, Healthy Recipes

Chapter Eight

Introduction to Recipes

If you've ever strolled through a health food store, you might feel as though you are in a foreign country when you see foods such as tempeh, millet, stevia and carob. You don't have to shop at a health food store to use this cookbook. For the most part, I have tried to make these recipes as tasty and delicious with foods from your local grocery store.

But for those people who have been shopping at a health food store already, or who need to find healthy alternatives due to conditions such as lactose intolerance from dairy, I have included some alternatives. For example, sea salt is a more nutritious salt than regular salt. Sucanat is a healthier type of brown sugar, and stevia is a natural replacement for artificial sweeteners. I have discussed various types of oils and vinegars in the salad dressing section, and more about soy products in the Tofu and Tempeh (chapter 18). A list of substitutes is included in Appendix D. Here is a short glossary of foods you might use from your health food store.

Arrowroot Powder: A starch made from a tropical root plant which makes an excellent substitute for cornstarch. (Cornstarch can cause digestive problems.) Used primarily as a thickening agent, it needs to be diluted in cold, not warm liquid so it won't be lumpy. It tends to add a shiny quality to sauces.

Braggs Amino Acids: A condiment for flavoring dressings, casseroles, soups, and other dishes which is very similar to soy sauce, but without the extra salt and fermentation. One tablespoon equals approximately one teaspoon of salt.

Carob Powder: The powder is made from the carob pods, which is a fruit that is high in minerals and low in fat. It tastes similar to chocolate, but not exactly. However, it can be a good substitute for chocolate in many recipes since it's naturally sweet and contains no caffeine. Chocolate needs a lot of sugar to be enjoyed.

Chapati: A flat, unyeasted bread common in India which is nice for dips or sandwiches.

Millet: A grain commonly familiar since it's been used in birdseed mixes for many years. Yet it's a wonderful, alkaline grain, easy to digest and great for people with wheat allergies. An ancient grain, it's commonly eaten in Africa and Asia. It's nice in stuffing and in place of rice in most dishes.

Sea Salt: Sun-dried and unrefined salt which contains no preservatives or bleaching agents found in refined salt. It also contains many trace minerals.

Shoyu: A type of soy sauce that contains more water than Tamari and is less condensed, but contains wheat. Tamari is wheat free. Both are used for flavoring foods.

Soba Noodles: A hearty, nutritious noodle made from buckwheat used often in Japanese dishes, commonly used in soups.

Soy Milk: Nutritious and delicious, soy milk is lactose/cholesterol-free yet high in Omega 3 fatty acids which can reduce cholesterol. Soy milk is high in protein and iron, and contains usable calcium. Use it cup-for-cup in place of milk for cooking. Vanilla flavor is nice for desserts and cereal. Read labels; some soy milks have as high as 10 grams of protein per serving. Soy ice cream and frozen yogurt are also available in most health food stores.

Soy Cheese: There are many varieties of soy cheeses made from soy milk so they are free from lactose and cholesterol. A small amount of casein is added to help it melt. TofuRella makes Cheddar, Jack, Mozzarella and Jalapeno styles. While not fat free, they are low in fat and high in protein. These cheeses are delicious. In my cooking classes, many students could not believe they ate tofu-based cheeses!

Stevia: Stevia is a naturally sweet herb that makes a good replacement for artificial sweeteners. Stevia is available in a dry powder form and also as a white or black liquid extract. So you may want to take color in consideration when you bake, since some liquids will darken your batter. Stevia can have an-almost licorice taste. Only 1 teaspoon is required to replace 1 cup of sugar. If you use stevia in place of honey, add more liquid to make up the difference. If you use it in place of a dry sweetener like sugar or Sucanat, add dry ingredients to make up the difference. (See pages 244-245.)

Sucanat: One of the most popular sweeteners, full of vitamins and minerals is Sucanat, made from evaporated sugarcane juice. Sucanat contains vitamins A and C, calcium, iron, potassium and chromium. Sucanat is far more natural than white sugar since it has far less processing. It has a mild taste similar to that of brown sugar and can be replaced for white sugar cup-for-cup. Sucanat Pure Cane Syrup is now available and is great for pancakes or baking.

Tamari: Tamari is a naturally fermented soy sauce without the added sugar or MSG found in other commercial soy sauces. It's naturally aged in wooden kegs for 2 years. Originally Tamari was a by product of the fermentation process of making miso. Tamari means wheat-free. It has a wonderful flavor and the reduced sodium type is available.

Tempeh: A soy food made from fermenting soybeans which makes a great meat substitute in foods such as enchiladas and vegetarian egg rolls. It has a chewy texture similar to pork. Tempeh is one of the highest sources of protein, and it's also predigested in a similar way as yogurt. Somewhat more nutritious than tofu, tempeh contain B12, and fiber. Tempeh needs to be flavored, and it makes a good meat extender. Tempeh can be sautéed or steamed and used in place of meat in egg rolls, cabbage rolls and similar dishes. Dried and ground, tempeh can substitute for ground nuts in recipes. It is often sold fresh or frozen in 8-ounce packages.

Tofu: A soybean curd made from cooking and straining soybeans and then coagulating them with nigari. Tofu is a great substitute for eggs, cottage, cheese and sour cream. It's high in protein, low in calories and contains no saturated fat or cholesterol. Tofu contains calcium, B vitamins and other minerals and is one of the most versatile of the soy foods and can be frozen, blended, marinated and mashed or used in dips, dressings, sauces, spreads, and desserts.

Yogurt Cheese: Real yogurt, made with live cultures is a good intestinal cleanser. When you use non-fat yogurt, yogurt cheese makes a good non-fat substitute for cheese, sour cream or cream cheese. Put the non-fat yogurt in a glass jar or container and let strain in a cheesecloth for 14 hours, preferably in the refrigerator. During the process, the whey will separate from the yogurt, leaving cheese. (See pages 99-100.)

About the Recipes

I wrote this book so people can shop at their local grocery store, or the health food store and still make these recipes. For example, you can substitute sea salt for salt, Tamari for soy sauce, and soy milk for milk in almost any recipe.

Most recipes in this cookbook serve 4 people.

Chapter Nine

Beverages

Smoothies, fruit juices, and herbal teas are all wonderful alternatives to beverages loaded with artificial sweeteners or chemicals. However, if you have a blood-sugar imbalance, I don't recommend drinking fruit drinks on a regular basis. For these people, eating the whole orange is better than drinking orange juice. But juices, especially freshly-squeezed juices are a better alternative to commercial sodas drinks. (See also chapter 26, Party Beverages and Desserts, page 222.)

Lemon Drink

Both a beverage and health tonic, this is a great way to start your morning. If you don't have an acid condition, lemons help the digestive system and are cleansing to the liver and bloodstream. You can substitute lemons for apple cider vinegar. (Using pasteurized lemon juice isn't as effective because using high temperatures kills natural enzymes, but it can still be used for taste.)

1 cup water

juice of one-half to 1 lemon (to taste)

Optional: 1 teaspoon honey or dash of Stevia

Drink hot or cold, but don't boil the lemon juice; add the lemon juice after heating the water.

Variation: 2 teaspoons apple cider vinegar in 1 cup water with 1 teaspoon honey.

Optional: A classic drink uses a dash of cayenne red pepper and raw maple syrup to stimulate digestion.

Healthy Lemonade

A great alternative to sugar-laden commercial lemonade.

1 cup lemon juice (juice from 3-4 lemons)
1 tablespoon honey or a few drops of Stevia liquid or
powder
5-6 cups of water

Blend ingredients well and serve or add ice.

Protein Drink

Wondering how to have a quick healthy breakfast? Try a quick breakfast drink with any of the soy protein powders available at health food stores. This is a good place to add one tablespoon of raw flaxseed oil or powder to get your quota of these protective Omega 3 fats.

One scoop of protein powder such as Nature's Plus
Spirutein or Designer Whey
1 cup of water, milk or soy milk
1 tablespoon flaxseed oil
Fruits as desired (banana, mango, pineapple, etc.)
Crushed ice

Put everything in a blender and blend for a minute.

Smoothies

Just about everyone loves smoothies, which is a term that suggests a blender drink somewhat like the milkshake that we all enjoy. They are quick, delicious, require few ingredients and taste great. Smoothies can be made with a mixture of all fruit, fruit and fruit juice, fruit and milk, or fruit and yogurt or tofu. Here are some varieties of each to choose from.

Fruits: *Fresh or frozen bananas, apples, strawberries, raspberries, papaya, blueberries, blackberries, or mangos.*

Sweetener: Choose a natural sweetener. Other sweeteners include dates, raisins, frozen fruit concentrates, maple syrup, honey, barley malt, brown rice syrup or stevia which are included in the glossary on natural sweeteners.

Liquid: Milk, tofu (flavored with vanilla and sweetener), non-fat yogurt, apple juice, pineapple juice, soy milk, rice milk, or almond milk.

Basic Smoothie

Here is a basic recipe that you can modify according to what you have available. If you use tofu in place of yogurt, be sure to get one that is a "silken" variety. Make just enough for your meal because smoothies lose their punch if they sit too long. They don't take long to make and you can make something different every day.

1 cup sliced fruit of choice

1 tablespoon honey or sweetener of choice

¼ teaspoon vanilla

1 to 1½ cups milk (or 8 ounces of non-fat yogurt, or silken tofu, or soy milk, or rice milk, etc.)

Crushed ice

Optional: 1 banana (omit if you are trying to lose weight.)

Optional: ½ teaspoon cinnamon for additional flavor
Blend all ingredients until creamy. Serve cold.

Variations:

For a Protein Drink Smoothie: Add 1 tablespoon protein powder
For an Orange Smoothie: Add 1-2 oranges
For Mocha Smoothie: Add 2 tablespoons Pero or coffee substitute
For Carob Smoothie: Add 1-2 tablespoons carob powder
For Peach Smoothie: Add 2 cups peaches
For Raspberry Smoothie: Add 1 cup raspberries

Fruit Slush

Slushes are great because they combine the fruit with the fruit drinks which adds more fiber. Slushes are fun drinks that can be enjoyed with a long ice tea spoon. They are nice for a party, too. I've made these drinks for a dinner party with my friend Michelle. Everyone loved the fresh taste and rated them high.

2 bananas

2 oranges

1 cup orange juice

1 cup pineapple juice

Crushed ice

Blend and serve cold. For variety, try other types of fruit. This is a good base for a protein drink, too.

Garnishes: Add lime wedge, strawberry wedge or pineapple wedge

Delightful Herbal Tea

I like to help my clients find healthier alternatives to caffeinated drinks. Finding a good herbal tea is helpful. Many of my clients like Celestial Seasonings Vanila Hazelnut, Almond Sunset, Mint Magic, and Bigelo's Lemon Ginger.

6 cups water

5-6 herbal tea bags

5-6 tablespoons honey (or stevia to taste)

¼ teaspoon ground cinnamon

½ cup fresh orange or lemon juice

Boil water and remove from heat. Add tea bags and brew for 5 minutes. Remove bags. Stir in honey, cinnamon and juices. Simmer again for 5 minutes.

Chapter Ten

Appetizers and Dips

Nearly every cuisine enjoys appetizers from Mexican Cheese Nachos to Mediterranean Humus Dip with Pita Bread. Some are so healthy and delicious, they make a wonderful mini meal. Below are some recipes I've made in cooking classes or just for friends.

Fresh Tomato Salsa

My students loved the taste of cherry tomatoes in this salsa which I created for one of my cooking classes.

12 cherry tomatoes or 3-4 ripe tomatoes, chopped

1 green onion, chopped

1 small onion, chopped

1 clove garlic, minced

2 tablespoons canned or fresh chilies

2 tablespoons parsley or cilantro

1 tablespoon vinegar (I prefer seasoned brown rice vinegar)

2 teaspoons lemon juice

½ teaspoon salt

Chop tomatoes, green onions and chilies. Mix all ingredients and chill. Serve with no-fat tortilla chips.

Variations: Add 1-2 teaspoon cumin and 1/4 teaspoon cayenne or 1 teaspoon chili powder. Or, add 1-2 ears of corn from the cob or 1 6-ounce can of corn, drained.

Low-Fat Tortilla Chips

Here's an easy way to make low-fat chips.

1 package corn tortillas

Seasoning of choice

Olive Oil or olive oil vegetable spray

Coat tortillas with vegetable spray or olive oil and place on a cookie sheet. Season with salt or Italian seasonings before baking. Cut corn tortillas into eighths. Bake in a 400° F. oven for 8-10 minutes. Serve with either salsa or bean dip.

Baked or Grilled Sweet Potato Chips

I made these one day when I was looking for a nice replacement for potato chips. The trick is to slice them as thinly as possibly and then season well. Even children enjoyed these chips.

2 sweet potatoes or yams, thinly sliced

Olive oil or Pam vegetable spray

¼ cup Parmesan cheese

½ teaspoon garlic salt (or ½ teaspoon Italian season-
   ings (I like Saltless Herbal Bouquet)

Spray a baking sheet with Pam spray or brush with olive oil. Lightly spray or brush sliced yams with olive oil and place on the baking sheet. Season and bake for 20 minutes at 400° F. Let cool and serve alone or with some type of creamy white dip.

Party Rye Sandwiches

This tasty spread goes so well on that dark, rich rye bread, often made in small party-size loafs. This recipe was another hit in my cooking classes.

3 tablespoons fat-free cream cheese, tofu, or tofu

 cream cheese

2 tablespoons Parmesan cheese

dash cayenne pepper

3 tablespoons minced onion

¼ teaspoon salt

1 tablespoon Dijon mustard

1 loaf party-size rye bread

Blend all ingredients except bread together. Spread on party-size rye bread and top with red pepper pieces. Bake at 350° F. for 5-10 minutes and serve warm.

Roasted Nut Mix

Nuts make a tasty substitute for a mixed nut snack. For variety, use chopped or slivered Brazil nuts, pine nuts, or sunflower seeds. (While nuts are a great fat, limit your serving sizes if you are trying to lose weight.)

2 tablespoons chopped almonds

2 tablespoons chopped cashews

2 tablespoons chopped pecans

2 tablespoons chopped walnuts

Soy sauce for flavor

Marinate the nuts almonds in enough soy sauce to cover. Drain nuts. Place in a non-stick pan or one sprayed with olive oil. Bake at 350° F. for 30-45 minutes or until nuts are dry and brown. Cool and serve as a snack.

Tasty Mini-Pizza

Pizza can be low-fat, quick and still healthy! Serenity Farm makes a delicious whole-wheat foccacia bread and coupled with Enrico's Pizza sauce makes a terrific pizza. (This recipe uses vegetables; add sliced chicken or other meat if desired.)

1 loaf Focaccia bread (or 1 package pita bread, sliced in half

1 8-ounce jar Pizza Sauce

1 teaspoon dried Italian seasoning

½ teaspoon salt

1 8-ounce package of low-fat Mozzarella cheese (or Parmesan cheese, grated)

½ cup thinly sliced onions

½ cup sliced mushrooms

1 red pepper, sliced in rings

Optional Toppings:

½ cup chopped each: sliced tomatoes or black olives

Spread the pizza or tomato sauce on the Foccacia bread or pita bread.* Sprinkle the Italian seasoning, and place the mushroom and onion slices on the bread. Place one red pepper ring over the onions and mushrooms. Add a few slices of tomatoes or black olives. Sprinkle with grated cheese. Place on a cookie sheet in a 350° F. oven and bake about 10-15 minutes until the cheese is melted and pizza is lightly browned around the edges.

(*If using pita bread, slice it in half and spread each half with sauce, seasoning, vegetables and cheese.)

Salmon and Cucumbers

This stuffing is versatile and can be used to stuff cucumbers, red peppers, tomatoes, or zucchini. I made it with canned salmon, but you can use fresh or canned tuna, (or even a vegetable filling like tempeh if you are adventurous). It's delicious and easy to make.

½ cup salmon (or tuna or grated tempeh)

1 cucumber, peeled (or vegetable of choice)

1 tablespoon mayonnaise

1 teaspoon grated onion

½ teaspoon lemon juice
Dash of pepper

Peel the cucumber and scoop out the center. Mash the fish and mix with the mayonnaise, onion, lemon juice and pepper. Stuff the cucumber and chill. Cut into ½" slices and serve.

Spinach Feta Mushroom Caps

1 tablespoon olive oil

1 tablespoon garlic, minced

1 large onion, minced

1 dozen large mushrooms (with caps separated and
   finely chopped)

1 10-ounce box frozen spinach, thawed and drained

¼ cup Feta cheese, crumbled

½ cup whole-wheat bread crumbs

In olive oil, sauté the onions, garlic and mushroom caps. (Put mushrooms aside.) Add the spinach and cook for 1-2 minutes. Place in a bowl and mix in the cheese and bread-crumbs. Fill the mushrooms and bake about 7-9 minutes in a 400° F. oven.

Garlic Mushrooms

Here's another delicious appetizer that's great for a party. Keep warm in oven if you like.

½ pound large stuffing mushrooms

1 cup leftover mashed potatoes or 8 ounces of blended tofu

1 clove garlic

1 teaspoon salt

2 tablespoons dried parsley

1 finely chopped green onion, minced

Wash and stem ½ pound large stuffing mushrooms. Combine mashed potatoes or tofu with garlic, parsley, green onion and salt. Fill mushroom caps. Lightly oil a shallow dish and bake at 350° F. for 15 minutes or until brown on top.

Stuffings and Dips

Dips can be low-fat and healthy. They add a serving of important beans or vegetables. Below are some ideas using vegetables, fish, tofu, yogurt, or various types of beans. In these recipes, yogurt and tofu can be used interchangeably.

How To Stuff Vegetables

One way to encourage your family to eat more vegetables is to serve them in a delicious, creative way. What do you stuff in these vegetables? Try bean dips, yogurt or tofu dips, grain dips, vegetable puree or dips, or whole-wheat bread crumbs.

Stuffed Tomatoes

Cut off tops and throw away. Scoop out pulp and invert tomatoes and drain on paper towel. Stuff with one of the dips listed later in this section.

Stuffed Zucchini

You may want to peel the zucchini first, especially if it's been sprayed with pesticides. Cut the top and bottom and cut in half. Remove the center seeds with a spoon and stuff with your favorite stuffing. You can leave these as long logs, or cut into shorter segments.

Stuffed Cabbage

Cabbage is easiest to stuff or roll when it's been slightly steamed (10 minutes). Place stuffing on end and roll, then roll left and right side toward center and fasten with a toothpick.

Stuffed Squash

The heavier squashes need to be slightly steamed before stuffing; the lighter squash, like yellow squash, just need to be peeled and cut in half. Then scoop out seeds and stuff.

Stuffed Mushrooms

Lightly wash and gently tear off the mushroom stems and use later or throw away. Place stuffing or dip in center of mushroom cap and add garnish if desired. Mushrooms can be served cold or hot.

Artichoke Heart Dip

This rich, flavorful dip is elegant enough for a special party, but simple enough for everyday. Be sure to blend until creamy. This was a hit in one of my cooking classes.

1 cup yogurt (or firm tofu)

1 6½-ounce jar artichoke hearts, drained

½ teaspoon Worcestershire sauce

2 tablespoon lemon juice

3 tablespoon whole-wheat bread crumbs

2 cloves garlic, minced

¼ teaspoon salt

Dash of cayenne pepper

½ pound mushroom caps, washed and stemmed

Put all ingredients except mushroom caps in a blender and blend until smooth. Stuff mushroom caps, or other vegetables.

Guacamole

1 ripe avocado (peeled, pitted)

3 tablespoons lemon juice

1 small tomato, chopped finely

1 small onion, chopped finely

1 teaspoon parsley flakes

½ teaspoon salt

1 garlic clove, minced

Mash avocado with lemon juice and stir in remaining ingredients. Serve with chips or vegetables.

Spinach Dip or Spread

1 10-ounce box frozen spinach, thawed

1 bunch leeks, chopped finely

1 8-ounce carton low-fat cream cheese (or tofu or cottage cheese)

1 tablespoon olive oil

1 clove garlic, minced

1 teaspoon dried basil

¼ teaspoon salt

¼ teaspoon white pepper

Place in food processor or blender and process until smooth. Use for crackers, vegetables or bread.

Fruit Dip

For that special menu when you want to serve fresh fruit with some pizzaz, try this easy-to-make dip. I served this as an appetizer for a dinner at Michelle's. I put the dip in a glass bowl in the center of a large glass plate. Arrange sliced bananas, red grape and green grapes around the dip.

1 cup yogurt or tofu

½ cup chopped dates

½ cup chopped raisins
Dash of vanilla

Optional: ¼ cup chopped figs

Blend well in blender. Chill and serve with a bowl of washed and cut-up fruits like bananas, strawberries and grapes.

Mediterranean Humus

Humus is a traditional Indian dip made from garbanzo beans and sesame seed butter or tahini. You can eliminate the sesame seed butter and make a delicious, low-fat dip.

1 cup cooked, drained garbanzo beans

  (or 1 16-ounce can)

½ cup lemon juice
2 cloves garlic, minced or ¼ teaspoon garlic powder

Dash of salt and cayenne pepper

¼ cup water
Parsley sprigs for garnish

Optional: 2 tablespoons tahini or sesame butter or 1 tablespoon olive oil.

Drain beans and pour into blender or food processor. Add spices and blend well until creamy consistency. Chill. Serve with chips, pita bread, chapati bread or vegetables.

Variations: Add 2 tablespoons Tamari soy sauce or ¼ teaspoon dried ginger root, or freshly grated ginger root. Also, try ½ cup chopped tomatoes or other spices like: cumin, coriander, or paprika. Garnish with parsley sprigs.

Spicy Black Bean Dip

My students liked the versatility of this dip since you can replace any bean recipe with black beans. Black beans make a traditional dip and when combined with corn chips, they make a complete protein snack.

2 cups cooked black beans, drained and mashed

1 teaspoon salt

¼ teaspoon coriander
Dash of cayenne pepper

3 cloves garlic, minced

2 tomatoes, chopped

Optional: ½ can sliced Jalapenos

Blend together by hand or in a food processor and chill. Serve with low-fat baked corn chips. Keeps about two weeks in the refrigerator and can be frozen.

Tofu Dill Dip

This tofu dip is a wonderful replacement for sour cream on a baked potato.

½ teaspoon garlic powder
2 tablespoons dried dillweed

2 tablespoons apple cider or brown rice vinegar

¼ cup olive oil
12 ounces tofu, firm

¼ teaspoon salt or sea salt
Dash of pepper

Blend really well in a blender until it's smooth. It's great with tortilla chips, raw vegetables, or baked potato chips.

Yogurt Cheese for Dips

Yogurt cheese is a popular, non-fat substitute for high-fat cheeses and makes wonderful dips and desserts. It can be substituted for ricotta cheese, cream cheese or tofu. I haven't seen yogurt cheese commercially available yet, but it's easy to make at home.

1 quart fresh non-fat, plain yogurt

Either use a yogurt cheese maker, or line a bowl with cheesecloth. Put yogurt in a bowl or yogurt cheese maker and gather ends of cheesecloth. Lift bag and allow liquid from the yogurt to drip into a bowl underneath. Tie both of the ends of cheesecloth on the refrigerator shelf and hang in a refrigerator approximately four hours. Remove cheesecloth.

Now you can flavor your "cheese" with your favorite herbs or: chives, garlic, dill (see dips below). Use in place of regular cheese, or in dips, sauces, salad dressings or desserts.

Drain for 4-6 hours for sour cream consistency.

Drain 12 hours or longer for whipped cream consistency.

Drain 24 hours or longer for cream cheese consistency.

Yogurt Cheese Onion Dip

This is a great substitute for the Lipton's Onion Dip that I used to make when I was growing up. It's low in fat, delicious and healthy.

8 ounces yogurt cheese (or substitute low-fat cottage cheese or tofu)

1-2 tablespoons apple cider vinegar

1 teaspoon dillweed

1 teaspoon garlic powder

1 teaspoon chili powder

1 onion, minced well

Combine spices with yogurt cheese in a blender and whirl until creamy. Served with raw cucumbers, carrot slices, broccoli flowerettes, celery stalks, or other vegetables. This dip is also nice with baked chips or whole-grain crackers.

Chapter Eleven

Savory Sauces

Sauces are fairly easy to make and add flavor to many simple foods. Below are two of my favorites made with healthy ingredients rather than artificial flavorings. More sauces are found in the pasta chapter which starts on page 196.

Easy Tomato Sauce

Quick and easy, oil is optional for this tomato sauce. Use lots of fresh tomatoes and spices for a rich tasting, low-fat sauce.

Vegetable spray or 1 teaspoon olive oil

1 onion, minced

1 clove garlic, minced

1 stalk celery, chopped

2 cups chopped tomatoes

2 tablespoons parsley flakes

Optional spices: 1 teaspoon each: basil and oregano

Sauté onion and vegetables in vegetable spray or oil. Add spices; bring to boil, and simmer 20 min. Serve warm over pasta or vegetarian entrees. You can add ground beef or ground tempeh, or Ready Ground Tofu, which is a commercially prepared tofu product which resembles ground hamburger, to any tomato sauce.

Hearty Spaghetti Sauce

For that special dinner that everyone will love, here's an even richer sauce:

1 tablespoon olive oil

½ onion, chopped

3 cloves garlic, minced

4 large tomatoes or 1 large can tomatoes

5 ounces of mushrooms, sliced

½ green pepper, chopped

1 can tomato paste

1 tablespoon parsley

1 teaspoon each: basil and oregano

Dash of cayenne

Salt, white pepper to taste

Sauté onion and garlic in oil. Stir in tomatoes and spices. Bring to boil, lower heat and simmer 15-20 minutes, or until thick.

Variation: Add 8 ounces ground turkey, grated tempeh or Ready Ground tofu and sauté with onions for added protein and texture.

Dijon Mustard Sauce (see Greek Lentils)

I originally created to encourage people to eat more lentils. But this sauce could be used over pasta, or even as a dip. To make entirely no-fat, omit the olive oil.

2 tablespoons Dijon mustard

½ teaspoon cumin

¼ teaspoon oregano

1 teaspoon salt or sea salt

Optional: 2 tablespoons olive oil

Blend well. Stir in with cooked beans (lentils or white beans work especially well), or pour over pasta.

Barbecue Sauce

Your own home-made healthy, barbecue sauce:

1 6-ounce can tomato paste

5-6 tablespoons red wine vinegar

1½ cups water

1 tablespoon Worcestershire sauce

½ onion, chopped

2 tablespoons brown sugar or Sucanat

1 teaspoon honey

1 teaspoon garlic powder

1 tablespoon chili powder

1 tablespoon Dijon mustard

1 tablespoon miso

1 teaspoon dried parsley

½ teaspoon salt

Combine all ingredients in a sauce pan. Bring to a low boil, reduce heat and simmer 15-20 minutes. Nice over meat loaf, chicken or anytime you want a barbecue sauce.

Pesto for Pasta

Pesto is a traditional Italian sauce for flavoring pasta made with pine nuts, basil and olive oil, it's a wonderful sauce for garlic and basil lovers. Here's my low-fat, healthy version.

2 tablespoons olive oil

Dash of salt

¼ cup dried basil, or ¾ cup fresh basil
2 cloves garlic, minced

½ cup almonds, chopped fine

Blend above ingredients well. Gently spoon in a sauce pan and heat until warm. Serve over cooked pasta.

Mock Alfredo Sauce

Blended tofu makes a wonderful, creamy sauce and is excellent as a replacement for high-fat cream in Alfredo Sauce. Here's a tasty version that your family will enjoy!

¼ onion, minced
1 clove garlic, minced or 1 teaspoon garlic powder

1 pound firm silken tofu

2 teaspoons soy sauce or Tamari

1 teaspoon dried basil

1 teaspoon salt or salt to taste

Spray a pan with 1 teaspoon olive oil and sauté onion and garlic until onions are limp. Put in a blender and blend together with tofu and spices. Gently warm in a saucepan for about 5 minutes in low heat. Serve over pasta.

Easy Gravy

This couldn't be easier and tastier.

1 cup water

2-3 tablespoons whole-wheat flour

1 tablespoon cornstarch or arrowroot powder

1 tablespoon soy sauce or Tamari

In cold water, combine cornstarch or arrowroot and whole-wheat flour and blend until dissolved. Then in a sauce pan, heat until it comes to a boil. Turn down heat and add Tamari sauce and serve over mashed potatoes.

Vegetable Sweet and Sour Sauce

A tangy oriental-type sauce with lots of flavor and little fat. Use this sauce to flavor noodles or pasta.

Vegetable spray

2 onions, chopped

1 green pepper, chopped

3 stalks celery, chopped

1 pineapple, cut in chunks (or 1 can), drained

4 tablespoons whole-wheat flour

4 cups water

4 tablespoons soy sauce or Tamari

Dash of salt or sea salt

Spray a pan with 1 teaspoon olive oil and sauté onions until they are translucent. Add green pepper, celery and pineapple and continue to sauté. In a separate bowl, combine salt and flour and water stirring well. Slowly pour flour mixture into vegetable mixture and stir well. Lower flame and simmer 10 minutes. Add soy sauce and simmer a few minutes. Serve over cooked noodles or pasta.

White Sauce

Here's a nice low-fat white sauce. Adding ¼ teaspoon of cayenne pepper gives it a little zip!

1 tablespoon cornstarch or arrowroot powder

1 cup water or chicken stock

2 tablespoons whole-wheat pastry flour

2 onions, steamed or boiled

2 potatoes, boiled

Dilute the arrowroot powder or cornstarch in liquid, add flour and stir. Puree the potatoes and onions and add to the cornstarch/flour mixture. Pour into a saucepan and stir until thick over medium heat, adding more liquid if necessary. Season with sea salt or cayenne.

Variation: Add ½ cup of grated tofu cheese and you have a great sauce for Macaroni and Cheese. Serve over broccoli or cauliflower. You can use this white sauce in place of all au gratin recipes.

Homemade Cranberry Sauce

A great addition to any Thanksgiving dinner, this homemade version is delicious. I made it for a Thanksgiving cooking class.

2 cups fresh or frozen cranberries

½ cup frozen apple juice concentrate

¾ cup brown sugar (or Sucanat or honey)

¼ to ½ cup chopped walnuts

1 teaspoon grated orange peel

Mix all ingredients together in a saucepan and bring to a boil. Lower heat and simmer for 5 to 10 minutes until berries pop. Remove from heat and refrigerate. Serve cold.

Chapter Twelve

Oils and Vinegars

Have you noticed that it's hard to eat a salad without a dressing? Salads are a great place to get your daily serving of the good essential fats. Salad dressings can be made with oil and vinegar, vegetable puree, milk, yogurt or a tofu base. Oil-based dressings traditionally use either lemon juice or vinegar plus some spices. Below are various types of herbs and spices, vinegars and oils commonly used in salad dressings.

Spices: Dill, curry, coriander, cumin, cayenne, Dijon mustard, ginger, garlic, horseradish, thyme, basil and mint. (see the Herbs and Spices in Appendix E on page 246.)

Sweeteners: Honey, maple syrup, stevia or frozen juice concentrates. (See the list of natural sugar substitutes in Appendix D on page 242.)

Glossary of Vinegars and Oils

Vinegars help digest high-protein foods. Naturally-brewed vinegars are preferred since distilling and heating destroys the beneficial enzymes. Vinegars should not be overly filtered and sometimes appear slightly cloudy.

Vinegars

Apple cider vinegar: One of the best vinegars for all-purpose use, apple cider vinegar is made from apples. It helps correct mineral balance and restores acid/alkaline balance. Purchase raw, unpasteurized apple cider vinegar which aids digestion, but is also excellent when used in salad dressings.

Brown rice vinegar: This is a slightly sweet, naturally brewed vinegar made from brown rice. Spectrum makes a nice seasoned brown rice vinegar that is so delicious that it requires no additional herbs.

Red wine vinegar: Red wine vinegar is rich, hearty and strong and can overpower some herbs. To substitute red wine vinegar when your recipe calls for a milder vinegar, simply use 1 or 2 tablespoons less. Spectrum also makes a nice herbal wine vinegar which is made from red wine vinegar. Eden's red wine vinegar is raw, unpasteurized and contains the healthy enzymes found in apple cider vinegar.

White wine vinegar: This is a mild, clear vinegar, for dishes that require mild flavoring.

Balsamic vinegar: For a richer taste use this semi-sweet vinegar made from white grapes, often aged in wooden casks for long periods of time for a richer taste.

Raspberry vinegar: A sweet, fruity vinegar flavored with raspberries. Often raspberry vinegar is used to make a wonderful raspberry tasting salad dressing.

Oils

Research proves that everyone needs some good oil in their diet. Lack of essential fatty acids (Omega 3, 6 and 9) can cause dry hair, brittle nails and dry skin. Essential oils are also protective against heart disease, cancer and diabetes. So a good place to get these oils is in your salad dressings.

Each tablespoon contains 14 grams of fat, so if you use 4 tablespoons (¼ cup oil) that's 56 grams of fat. Reduce the recipe even further if you want to reduce the fat. Only using one or two tablespoons will often carry the flavor and still give you those essential fatty acids.

Unfortunately, many of the oils that are available at the grocery store have been solvent extracted or damaged. I don't recommend an oil unless it says on the label that it was cold or expeller pressed. If it doesn't say how it was processed, it was probably processed with harmful chemicals.

(See *Why Can't I Lose Weight?* for more information.) Olive oil is the safest oil to purchase in the grocery store. The rest are best purchased from your health food store, but I would recommend that you still check the label for the term cold-pressed.

Corn: Use with medium heat cooking. Corn oil tastes best in whole-grain baked goods.

Olive: Made from olives, extra virgin, virgin and pure. An incredibly healthy oil used for centuries throughout the world. Can be used for baking or stir-frying.

Canola: A great all-purpose oil, especially nice for sautéing and in salads or baking.

Safflower and Sunflower: Use with low-heat cooking or for salad dressings.

Sesame: A delicious oil especially nice for oriental type dishes; one of the few oils that can be heated to high enough temperature to stir-fry.

Flaxseed: One of the best sources for Omega 3 fatty acids, flaxseeds can be ground, or purchased in capsules. Barlean's,

Rohe, Spectrum and Arrowhead Mills all make flaxseed oil and other products.

German nutritionist Dr. Johanna Budwig has done excellent research on flaxseed oil reporting how protective it is against certain types of cancer and for lowering cholesterol levels. Flaxseed oil should *only* be used as a salad dressing or in a protein blender drink since heating will damage it.

Walnut and Almond: Both can be used for gourmet-type dishes when you want an elegant or unusual taste.

Chapter Thirteen

Super Salad Dressings

Salad dressings can be as basic as equal parts of lemon juice and olive oil with a dash of salt, and some herbs and spices. Let's begin with a basic vinaigrette and add variations. These dressings can be made in a blender, or a jar with a lid for shaking.

Basic Italian Vinaigrette Dressing

A simple yet elegant Italian dressing.

¼ cup extra virgin olive oil

¼ cup lemon juice

1 clove garlic, minced

Dash of salt

Optional: 1 teaspoon each: marjoram, oregano and basil

Blend well and serve.

Creamy Vinaigrette

2 tablespoons olive oil

2 tablespoons lemon juice or 4 tablespoons vinegar

1 teaspoon Dijon mustard

1 teaspoon basil

Dash of salt or salt to taste

¾ cup plain non-fat yogurt

Blend well and serve.

Variations: If you get tired of the same flavor every day, you'll be glad to try the variety of herbs that are available. Here are several variations on a basic vinaigrette. Add any one of the following:

1 clove garlic

1 teaspoon each dill and caraway

1 teaspoon coriander and cumin

1 teaspoon thyme and basil

2 teaspoons poppy seeds

1 teaspoon each: garlic and basil

1 teaspoon each: savory and marjoram

1 teaspoon each: paprika, basil, marjoram and rosemary

1 teaspoon each: basil, parsley, marjoram, rosemary

1 teaspoon each: basil, oregano, marjoram, garlic, sage and thyme

1 teaspoon cayenne

Sweet dressing: Add one of the following: 1 teaspoon honey or 3 tablespoons frozen orange juice concentrate.

Curry dressing: Add one of the following: ¼ cup oil; ¼ cup vinegar; 1 teaspoon cumin; 1 teaspoon coriander; 1 teaspoon turmeric; or ¼ teaspoon cayenne.

No-oil Italian Dressing

It's possible to make a salad dressing without any fat or oil. Just use more herbs and vinegar. Here's a good no-fat dressing.

¼ cup lemon juice

¼ cup apple cider vinegar

¼ cup apple juice

½ teaspoon each: oregano, garlic powder, rosemary, basil, sage and onion

Mix together in a blender and serve.

Tofu Dijon Dressing

Tofu makes a creamy, rich dressing. Here's a nice tofu dressing that can be used as a dip, too.

16 ounces firm tofu

2 tablespoons vinegar

1 tablespoon Dijon mustard

1 tablespoon olive oil

1 teaspoon lemon juice

1 clove garlic, minced

¼ cup water

Combine in a blender and blend at low speed. This will last about a week in the refrigerator.

Avocado Dressing

Avocados are a rich source of Omega 3 fatty acids, the good type of fat which is essential to our health. This dressing is healthy, but needs to be eaten in moderation.

2 medium avocados

1 green onion

1 clove garlic

Pinch of cayenne

Dash of salt

1 teaspoon lemon juice

2 tablespoons water

Combine ingredients in a blender and blend until smooth.

Variation: Add ½ cup green onion, chopped

Healthy Thousand Island

This is easy to make, and tastes just like the original. It's low in fat, too. I like to use Spectrum Lite Canola Mayonnaise.

¼ cup mayonnaise (I like Tofu Nayonaise)

3 tablespoons ketchup

2 tablespoons lemon juice

¼ cup dill pickle, chopped fine
Blend and serve.

Ranch Dressing

A healthy, low-fat version of a formerly high-fat dressing. I made this with tofu at Michelle's dinner party, but yogurt makes it even creamier. Enjoy!

½ onion, minced

1 cup plain yogurt

½ cup vinegar

4 teaspoons Dijon mustard

2 teaspoons Sucanat or honey

4 cloves garlic, minced

4 tablespoons olive oil

½ teaspoon oregano
Combine ingredients in a blender and blend well until smooth.

Chapter Fourteen

Lucious Salads

Eating one or two salads a day is a great way to get your "five a day" servings of fruits and vegetables. Green salads are wonderful and can be made from a variety of greens: Boston, bib, Chinese cabbage, red and green cabbage, loose leaf red and green lettuce, chard, watercress, kale, romaine or spinach.

A basic salad could include vegetables such as chopped celery, carrots, green pepper, tomatoes, celery or cucumber. For variety, you can make bean salads by combining cooked beans with a salad dressing, grains, or pasta, combining the ingredients with vegetables.

Classic Mixed Green Salad

Here's a classic green salad, perfect for lunch or dinner salad.

1 head chopped green leaf lettuce

1 head chopped Romaine lettuce

3-4 shredded carrots

1 red pepper, sliced

Other favorite salad vegetables

Dressing: Make your own from a good quality vegetable oil like olive oil or flaxseed oil, or buy a salad dressing that does not contain hydrogenated oils like Spectrum or Arrowhead Mills (found at specialty shops or health food stores). Another idea is to use avocado or salsa for dressing.

Greek Salad

Another hit in my cooking classes! This is a delicious beautiful salad that's flavored well. Use the special dressing or a vinaigrette.

1 bunch red leaf or green leaf lettuce, torn in small pieces

1 small cucumber, cut in chunks

1 red pepper, cut in chunks

½ cup black olives, cut lengthwise (optional)

1 small white onion, chopped fine

2 small Roma tomatoes

Wash and peel cucumber and chop vegetables. Toss ingredients together and serve with dressing.

Dressing:

2 tablespoons olive oil

2 tablespoons lemon juice

2 cloves garlic, minced

1 teaspoon each: salt, parsley, and paprika

½ teaspoon basil

2 teaspoons oregano

Dash of cayenne

Mix ingredients and blend. Pour over salad and garnish with black olives or Feta cheese.

Grilled Chicken Caesar Salad

Eating a salad with some protein makes a perfect start for a meal. Serve with a slice of whole-grain bread.

Dressing:

1 clove garlic (minced fine, pressed or crushed)

3 tablespoons Spectrum olive oil

2 tablespoons lemon juice

1 teaspoon Dijon mustard

Dash of salt or salt substitute

Salad:

1 head Romaine lettuce

6-8 strips of grilled chicken

1 cup garlic croutons (see recipe below)

Parmesan cheese

Mix garlic, oil, lemon juice, mustard and salt in a bowl. Wash and dry lettuce and break into bite-size pieces. Add chicken strips, and toss. Top with Parmesan cheese and garlic croutons.

Crouton recipe: 1 slice whole-wheat toast: 1 tablespoon Spectrum olive oil or Pam spray, 1 clove garlic, whole-wheat bread slices. Rub both sides of toast with clove of garlic and gently brush oil or spray with Pam. Keep warm. Cube and toss in salad.

Most meat markets or grocery stores carry prepared grilled chicken strips.

Mexican Taco Salad

Another healthy version of a favorite salad. Two spice combinations available that I like are: Hain Taco Seasoning Mix and Santa Fe Taco Mix. Both can be used with either beef, chicken, turkey or tempeh. If you want to make your own seasoning mix, combine equal parts of chili, garlic, basil, cumin, oregano, ginger, parsley and cayenne. My friend Susan Brooks made this recipe with chicken and said it was delicious. Using grated tempeh makes it a low-fat salad.

8 ounces ground beef, chicken, turkey or tempeh (if using tempeh, grate and sauté it with 1 teaspoon each chili powder and oregano)

½ medium onion

1 package taco seasoning mix

1 head green leaf lettuce

½ cabbage, shredded

1 16-ounce can kidney beans, drained

3 carrots, chopped

1 tomato, chopped

¼ cup cheddar cheese, grated (or soy cheese)

Sauté ground meat and add onion, Taco seasoning mix and water. Mix and cook, stirring 5-10 minutes. Meanwhile, combine cabbage, kidney beans, carrots, and tomatoes in a large bowl. Cover with Taco seasoning mixture and top with cheese.

Dressing Variation: Combine 2 tablespoons olive oil, ¼ cup brown rice vinegar, 1 teaspoon chili powder, and 1 teaspoon cumin. Blend well and pour over salad.

Dijon Tofu "Eggless" Salad

Here is a classic tofu egg salad. Most people don't even know it's made with tofu. I like using a firm tofu.

16 ounces firm tofu

1 onion, chopped

1 clove garlic, minced

2 tablespoons Dijon mustard

2 stalks celery

1 bunch leek, minced

2 tablespoons olive oil

2 tablespoons apple cider vinegar

Dash of salt and cayenne pepper

Chop vegetables. Crumble tofu with your hands and combine with vegetables. Mix Dijon mustard, oil and vinegar and pour over mixture. Stir well and serve. Serve as it is or refrigerate and serve cold. This salad makes a great stuffing for tomatoes, green or red peppers, stuffed in pita bread, or rolled in whole-wheat flour tortillas.

Option 1: For curry egg salad add 3 teaspoons curry powder.

Option 2: Blend tofu egg salad and add 1 teaspoon coriander and salt to taste. Makes a great curry dip.

Taboulie Salad

This was a real hit in the cooking classes. Taboulie is a traditional Middle Eastern salad, made with bulgur or cracked wheat, tomatoes, olive oil and sometimes mint. You can make a taboulie-type dish with cooked brown rice or millet too. Here's my version.

1 cup cracked wheat

1 cup hot water

4 tablespoons dried or ½ cup fresh parsley, chopped

2 green onions, minced

2 tablespoons olive oil

2 tablespoons lemon juice

Dash of salt and pepper

3-4 small Roma tomatoes, chopped

Combine cracked wheat and water and soak until water is well absorbed 45 minutes. Add remaining ingredients except tomato and mix well. Add tomatoes, chill and serve on a bed of lettuce or in a taco shell.

Almond Brown Rice Salad

This salad is delicious and especially nice for special occasions and entertaining!

2 cups cooked brown rice

½ onion, chopped fine

2 stalks celery, chopped fine

½ tomatoes, chopped

½ cup sliced almonds

½ cup seasoned brown rice vinegar or
**   brown rice vinegar, or white wine vinegar**

2 tablespoons olive oil

½ teaspoon each: cumin, basil and dill

In a salad bowl, combine rice, onions, celery, tomatoes and almonds. Separately make a dressing of brown rice vinegar, olive oil and spices. Combine well and serve.

Variations: You can substitute quinoa, corn grits or millet for rice.

Note about vinegars: Red wine and apple cider vinegars are very strong generally; and white wine or brown rice vinegars are milder. You could simply use apple cider vinegar in any of these recipes; however, for recipes that call for a milder vinegar, simply use less of the stronger vinegars.

Healthy Low-Fat Waldorf Salad

I used to really enjoy my Aunt Jerrie's Waldorf Salad she served at our family gatherings. Here's an updated version of this favorite:

2 medium-sized tart apples (Gravenstein), peeled and chopped

4 tablespoons dark raisins

5-6 tablespoons walnuts or sunflower seeds, chopped

1 stalk celery, chopped

Dressing:

½ cup yogurt

1 teaspoon lemon juice

2 teaspoons honey

Combine apples, raisins, seeds, and celery in a bowl. Mix dressing and pour over salad. Serve chilled.

Carrot Raisin Salad

Carrot salads are a great way to get kids to eat their carrots. Adding raisins and nuts makes it really special!

½ cup each raisins and walnuts

1 cup grated carrots

¼ cup lemon juice

2 tablespoons fructose

3 tablespoons plain yogurt

2 tablespoons oil

4 green or red lettuce leaves

Mix together all ingredients. Serve on green lettuce leaves.

Salad Nicoise

It's easy to omit the egg and substitute the tuna to get a nice healthy version of this traditional French salad.

¼ cup olive oil

2 tablespoons apple cider vinegar

1 teaspoon Dijon mustard

1 head Boston or Romaine lettuce

1 can tuna, drained

1 cup green beans

4 tomatoes, sliced

4 boiled eggs

Combine the oil, vinegar and mustard for the dressing. in a bowl; then combine vegetables and toss.

Lucious Fruit Salad

Want to make your own fruit salad cup—you know, the kind you used to get for lunch in your high school cafeteria— only this one is fresh, tasty and nutritious!

1 orange, peeled and sliced

1 grapefruit, peeled and sliced

½ fresh pineapple, peeled and sliced

1 papaya, peeled and slices

1 cup seedless grapes

Mix well and sprinkle ¼ cup orange juice over fruit and serve.

Optional: ¼ cup chopped almonds or walnuts

Chapter Fifteen

Vegetable Entrees

Vegetables are wonderful foods. They are highly nutritious, containing many vitamins, minerals and fiber. It's good to have a variety of above-the-ground (lettuce) and below-the-ground, (root vegetables). Generally, the harder, starchier vegetables need to be cooked, steamed, stir-fried, baked, or roasted. Softer vegetables can be eaten raw in salads. Vegetables combine nicely with meats, cheese, beans or grains. They make nice purees, spreads, soups, casseroles, sauces, and even desserts.

Washing vegetables: Fill your sink with cold water and add 4 tablespoons of salt and ½ cup vinegar or the juice from 2-3 lemons. Soak the fruits and vegetables for ten minutes and rinse under cold water. You can also use bleach. Use one tablespoon of bleach per gallon of water. Let your produce sit for 10 minutes; drain and rinse in clear water for 10 minutes. Bleach eliminates food sprays, bacteria, parasites, giardia, and other microbes.

Stir-frying is one of the tastiest ways to get your vegetables. Traditional stir fries often contain hydrogenated vegetable oils and monosodium glutamate (MSG). A healthier way to make a stir-fry is with olive oil and natural seasonings. Here are some different combinations of vegetable stir-fries that are found in the frozen department of most grocery stores.

Hunan: Broccoli, water chestnuts, carrots, and red pepper.

Bejan: Broccoli, water chesnuts, carrots, red pepper, pea pods, onions, sprouts, mushrooms, bamboo shoots, and celery.

Peking: Broccoli, carrots, red peppers, green beans, peas, and onions.

Lo Mein: Carrots, celery, red pepper, onion, broccoli, water chestnuts, and pea pods.

Mandarin: Broccoli, carrots, onions, pea pods, red pepper, mushrooms, bamboo shoots, and leeks.

I like using these colorful combinations since they also guarantee a wider variety of minerals and vitamins.

Steamed Vegetables

Quickly steaming vegetables makes them easier to digest, but still keeps their flavor.

1 bunch broccoli, chopped

2 tomatoes, quartered

1 red pepper, sliced

5-6 carrots and/or celery, sliced on diagonal

Bring 1 cup of water to a boil and steam the heartier vegetables first for 5-10 minutes (broccoli and carrots). Add the lighter vegetables next: tomatoes, red pepper, and celery and steam another 5 minutes. Try different combinations depending on the season and experiment with pasta sauces or just some olive oil with seasonings like garlic, cayenne or ginger.

Options: Try any of the stir-fry combinations listed above. Choose from: Hunan, Bejan, Lo Mein, Peking, or Mandarin. (See Vegetable Oriental Stir-fry on page 127.)

Vegetable Chop Suey

My students in the cooking classes loved this simple, delicious and healthy dish. You can make it a meal by adding chicken.

Sauce:

¾ cup vegetable broth

1 tablespoon soy sauce (or Tamari)

1 teaspoon honey

1 teaspoon brown rice vinegar or vinegar

1 tablespoon cornstarch diluted in 3 tablespoon water

Vegetables:

1 small onion, sliced in crescent shapes

½ cup celery, diagonal sliced

½ cup green cabbage, sliced or grated

1 cup mushrooms, sliced

1 green pepper, sliced diagonally

2 carrots, sliced on diagonal

½ cup water chestnuts

Combine ingredients for sauce in a bowl and set aside. Meanwhile, chop vegetables and lightly sauté in a saucepan sprayed with vegetable spray, or "water sauté" by adding ¼ cup water and stirring over low heat. Start with onions and add celery, cabbage, carrots, mushrooms, green peppers and water chestnuts in that order. When vegetables are still slightly crisp add the sauce mixture and simmer 10-15 minutes until sauce is slightly thick. Serve over cooked brown rice, cooked brown rice noodles or cooked Oriental noodles. For cooking noodles follow the recipe on package.

Roasted Garlic

Roasting garlic is a great way to use garlic. Roasting makes it creamy so it's great as a spread over rye or wheat crackers.

2 heads of garlic, unpeeled

Cut the top off (the pointed end) and brush with olive oil. Place in a baking dish in a 350° F oven. Bake 30-40 minutes until garlic is tender. Peel the garlic and use as a spread or as you would butter. Season to taste.

Vegetable Oriental Stir-fry

This is a delicious way to get your family to eat more vegetables. You can serve it with your choice of meat. If you are in a hurry, use frozen vegetables.

½ head cabbage or Chinese cabbage, shredded

4 onions, 4 stalks celery, 2 carrots, diagonally sliced

1 stalk broccoli, chopped

1 cup each: pea pods and water chestnuts

2 cloves garlic, minced

1 cup bean sprouts

Olive oil or Pam Olive Oil Spray

¼ cup soy sauce or Tamari

2-3 tablespoons cornstarch or arrowroot powder dissolved in 1½-2 cups water

Spray pan with Pam olive oil spray and add all the vegetables except for the sprouts and garlic and cook quickly until tender over lower heat about 5 minutes. At the last minute stir in the bean sprouts and garlic. Separately mix corn starch or arrowroot powder and water. Add to vegetables and stir over low heat. Add soy sauce or Tamari and serve.

Hot and Spicy Marinated Vegetables

The marinade flavors these vegetables nicely.

½ cup broccoli flowerets

½ cup carrots, sliced on diagonal

½ cup cauliflower flowerets

¼ cup red pepper, chopped

Dash of salt

Marinade: Mix together: ¼ cup olive oil, ¼ cup brown rice vinegar, ¼ teaspoon garlic powder, ¼ teaspoon chili powder, and a dash of sea salt. Lightly steam vegetables. Pour marinade over vegetables and toss gently. Cover and let sit for 15-30 minutes. Toss again and serve warm or cold.

Garlic Roasted Potatoes

You will love this mouth-watering dish!

3-4 potatoes, peeled and chopped

2 tablespoons olive oil

1 teaspoon rosemary

3-4 garlic cloves, minced

2 tablespoons of water

Combine ingredients and bake at 350° F. for 1 hour. Serve as a side dish.

Italian Mashed Potatoes

My class really liked the oregano flavor in these potatoes. Still delicious, still creamy, but low fat!

4-6 medium-sized white potatoes cut in round slices

1 can evaporated skim milk (or soy or rice milk)

1 tablespoon olive oil

Dash of white pepper, salt, and oregano

Boil potatoes until tender. Drain. Mash with fork and add oil and milk gradually with a mixer. Add spices and serve with parsley and gravy (See Easy Gravy recipe on page 106.) For creamier potatoes, add ½ cup blended tofu or yogurt to potatoes

Mashed Sweet Potatoes

Creamy, sweet and low-fat, but good enough for a pie filling if you add ¼ cup honey.

2 large sweet potatoes or yams, peeled and sliced

¼ cup low-fat yogurt or tofu

Dash of cinnamon

¼ cup orange juice concentrate

Cook potatoes 15 minutes or until tender. Mash with rest of ingredients. Serve warm.

Green Beans with Almonds and Baby White Onions

A great combination—even children will eat these vegetables.

2 pounds fresh green beans

1 cup raw slivered almonds

8 ounces baby white onions (raw or canned)

1 tablespoon lemon juice

¼ cup olive oil

¼ teaspoon salt

Cut the ends off the beans and steam them. Drain. Mix together lemon juice, oil and salt. Add mixture to the beans. Add almonds and onions, toss and serve.

Chapter Sixteen

Lean Bean Dishes

Beans are a wonderful addition to any diet, especially for vegetarians. Beans are highly nutritious, and low in fat, salt and sugar. They are a great source of vegetable protein, and combined with whole grains, they make a complete protein, comparable to animal proteins. They are one of the best sources of fiber, both soluble and insoluble. Beans are particularly good for diabetics, and are helpful for people with colon problems, high-blood cholesterol and high-blood pressure. However, it's important to take digestive enzymes if you are not used to eating beans (see page 132).

Beans can be used in chili, for dips, salads, soups, spreads, and with grains. There are many varieties of beans ranging from easy-to-cook red lentils which only take about 35 minutes to heartier soy beans which take 4-6 hours.

Flavoring and Using Beans

1. Rinse dry beans several times, until water is clear, removing any small stones. Soak beans overnight or for several hours (except for lighter lentil and split pea family). Soaking causes less gas since the sugars that tend to give people gas are water soluble and can be minimized by soaking. You can quick soak by boiling the beans 2 minutes and letting them stand an hour. Always discard the soaking water before cooking beans.

2. Smaller beans such as lentils, split peas, and aduki beans cook quickly. They don't need to be soaked, and they

can be cooked the same way as larger beans, but they only have to simmer for 30 minutes.

3. To determine if beans are soaked well enough, cut the bean in half. If the inside is lighter in color than the rest, the bean is undersoaked. A properly soaked bean is uniform in color.

4. Cook 1 cup of beans to approximately 4-5 cups of water. Bring water to a boil, add beans and simmer for 1½ hours or until tender. Do not overcook beans or allow the water to boil more than 10 minutes. Beans should be tender but firm. Garbanzo and Great Northern Beans must be simmered for at least 2-3 hours.

5. Try adding a piece of kombu seaweed to your cooking water to help decrease difficulties with digestion. Kombu is a seaweed which helps alkalize beans, adds minerals and makes beans easier to digest. Often kombu dissolves during cooking but if not, this piece can be removed later or chopped up and eaten. Another suggestion is to add 1 teaspoon of miso paste or 1 teaspoon of fennel seeds to the beans after they are cooked. Certain spices will also aid in digestion: ginger, garlic, cayenne and cumin.

6. Do not add salt or vinegar to the beans until they are cooked, as this will make them tough and prevents them from softening properly. To see if a bean is cooked enough, put a bean in your mouth and try to break it with your tongue. If it's done, you can mash it with your tongue; if not, it will be hard. Also, another indication is that some of the beans will have split their skins. However, too many split skins means you have overcooked the beans. Just eating a bean may be the best indicator. They should be tender, but not mushy.

7. Canned beans are actually a healthy food and are incredibly convenient. Canned beans are easier to digest than beans made from scratch because they are well cooked and

well seasoned with salt which improves their digestibility. For that reason, I usually drain and rinse the beans before using them. Most of the recipes in this cookbook can be prepared with either home cooked or canned beans.

There are several varieties (Eden, Westbrae) that are low in salt and fat, and come in lead-free cans.

8. Many people who change over to a more vegetarian diet have difficulty digesting beans. That's because we often lack enzymes to help break down bean sugars before they reach the intestines. Some products like Beano and Say Yes to Beans both help. Add a few drops to the first spoonful. Beano and other bean enzymes also assist in digesting foods such as cabbage and cauliflower. To get your digestive system accustomed to digesting beans, eat small quantities at a time, and try to eat them consistently, a few times every week. Sprouted beans seem to be the most digestible, since the starch has already begun to convert to sugar. Most sprouts can be eaten raw, however, soy bean sprouts need to be cooked first.

To Soak or Not

Soft beans like green and red lentils, split peas and mung beans require no soaking and take the shortest amount of time, varying from 30-45 minutes.

Medium beans like aduki, pinto, kidney, navy, black, lima need to be soaked. They are usually cooked in 2 hours.

Large hard beans like garbanzos, soy beans, and other large beans need to be soaked overnight and cooked for at least 4 hours.

Cooking Beans

One Cup	Water	Cooking Time	Yield
Aduki	3 cups	2 hours	2 cups
Anasaki	3 cups	90-120 minutes	2 cups
Black	3-4 cups	60-90 minutes	2 cups
— Black-eyed			
Peas	3 cups	45-60 minutes	2 cups
Fava Beans	2 cups	90-120 minutes	2 cups
Garbanzo	4 cups	90-120 minutes	2 cups
Great Northern			
Beans	3½ cups	60-90 minutes	2 cups
Kidney	3 cups	60-90 minutes	2 cups
Lentils	3 cups	30-45 minutes	2¼ cups
Lima	2 cups	60-90 minutes	1¼ cups
Mung	3 cups	60 minutes	2 cups
Navy	3 cups	90-120 minutes	2 cups
— Pinto	3 cups	90-120 minutes	2 cups
Red	3 cups	2 hours	2 cups
Split peas	3 cups	30 minutes	2¼ cups
Soy Beans	4 cups	4-6 hours	2 cups

Flavoring Beans

One of the first concerns with bean cooking is how to get a good flavor without the fat from the lard, ham and ham bones. You can still bake flavorful beans without added fat. Instead of using just plain water, add vegetable broth, chicken broth, or vegetable bouillon to cook the beans.

For flavoring beans after they are cooked, use naturally fermented soy sauce (Tamari), Miso, or Bragg's amino acids. (See glossary on pages 82-85.)

For spicy beans: Use a bay leaf, cayenne, garlic and onions.

For Italian style beans: Use Italian seasoning mix, lemon pepper, or curry powder.

For black beans: Use cumin, sea salt and cayenne.

For Boston baked beans: Use 4-5 teaspoon Sucanat, ¼ cup molasses, 1 teaspoon Dry mustard, ½ teaspoon white pepper.

For legumes: Use paprika, thyme, or oregano.

To thicken beans: Use one potato or dry potato flakes, oatmeal, oat bran, or blended tofu.

Greek Lentils

This is one of my students' favorite dishes. These herbs and spices make a great dish or side dish. You could even add pasta to make a Greek Lentil Pasta Salad.

1 cup dried lentils

2 tablespoons Dijon mustard

¼ teaspoon oregano

½ teaspoon cumin

2 tablespoons olive oil

1 onion, minced

1 teaspoon salt

Optional: ripe olives, Feta cheese

Wash and rinse lentils. Add 2 cups of water and bring to a boil. Cover and simmer for 30 minutes. Cool. In a separate bowl, combine spices and stir well. Pour over lentils and mix well. These lentils can be served hot or cold.

Variation: Add 1 cup cooked pasta to make a pasta-lentil salad. Make a Greek Taco by using this mixture on a corn or flour tortilla.

Refried Beans

A traditional Mexican dish, only without the added lard!

3 cups dried pinto beans, soaked

6 cups water

1 bay leaf

1 carrot

1 teaspoon salt

3 medium onions, chopped

3 tablespoons extra-virgin olive oil

1 teaspoon dried oregano

1 teaspoon dried basil

1 tablespoon ground cumin

Optional: Tabasco or hot sauce

Drain beans. Place in a large pot and cover with 1 inch of water. Add bay leaf and carrot and bring to a boil. Reduce heat and simmer 45 minutes, covered. Add the salt and cook 10 more minutes. Remove carrot and bay leaf. Drain the beans, reserving the cooking liquid.

Sauté the onions in olive oil for about 8 minutes, or until soft. Add the oregano, basil and cumin and continue to sauté 5 more minutes, adding ¼ cup of the bean liquids. Add the beans and mash to a thick paste. Cook over low heat, uncovered, for about 8 minutes, adding bean liquid as necessary. Season and serve.

Spicy Black Beans

A delicious black bean dish.

½ teaspoon olive oil

1 small onion, minced

1 clove garlic, minced

4 carrots, chopped

2 cans black beans drained (or cooked from scratch)

1 cup corn, drained

1 teaspoon salt

½ teaspoon cumin

¼ teaspoon white pepper

Sauté onion and garlic in oil or vegetable spray. Add carrots and sauté until tender. Add black beans, corn, and seasonings. Cook until heated through, about 5 minutes. Serve with brown rice and a salad.

Honey Baked Beans

2 cups dried navy beans

1 teaspoon ginger

1 medium onion, chopped

2 tablespoons honey

¼ cup brown sugar or Sucanat

1 teaspoon salt

1 teaspoon Dijon mustard

4-5 cups of bean liquid (or water)

Sort and wash beans and soak for 3 hours. Rinse beans, cover with water and simmer (below boil) in a covered saucepan for 1 hour. Drain beans, reserving 3 cups of liquid. In a separate bowl, combine the bean liquid, ginger, onion, honey, salt and mustard. Mix with beans and place beans in a baking dish. Cover with foil and bake in 300° F oven for 3-4 more hours. Stir occasionally. (For even richer tasting beans, add ¼ cup molasses.)

Spanish Garbanzo Beans

For variety, here's a Spanish style bean dish. They are great!

6 cups cooked garbanzo beans

8 tomatoes, chopped

2 onions, chopped

2 green peppers, chopped

2 teaspoons each: oregano, basil, celery seed

1-2 cloves garlic, chopped

Combine ingredients and cook until flavors are combined and vegetables are tender.

Mediterranean Tacos

Here's another version of Mediterranean Humus.

8-10 whole-grain flour tortillas

1 cup cooked garbanzo beans

½ teaspoon cumin

2 cloves garlic

2 teaspoons lemon juice

½ teaspoon salt

Dash of cayenne pepper

Optional: ¼ teaspoon sesame buter or tahini

Blend all ingredients except tortillas and place on a whole-grain flour tortilla. Top with shredded lettuce, chopped tomatoes, onions, cucumbers and sprouts.

Vegetarian Enchiladas

These are great! Easy-to-fix and delicious, they were another hit in the cooking classes.

8-10 corn or flour tortillas

Olive oil spray

Filling:

2 cups cooked pinto beans

16 ounces tofu, mashed

½ teaspoon ground cumin

2 cloves garlic, minced

1 onion, chopped

Optional: ½ can sliced Jalapenos

Dash of salt

Combine all ingredients for the filling together in a blender and lightly blend 1 or 2 minutes (still chunky).

Enchilada Sauce:

1 can tomato paste

4-5 teaspoons chili powder

¼ teaspoon each: oregano, cumin, garlic and onion powder

2 cups water (or more as needed)

2 tablespoons corn meal

Combine together in a saucepan and cook for 10 minutes.

To assemble enchiladas: Spray a 9 x 13-inch baking dish with olive oil spray. First, lightly dip tortillas one at a time in the sauce and fill each one with approximately 2 tablespoons of filling. Roll up and place in a baking dish, next to each other. Continue to fill each one until the filling and tortillas are used. Cover with enchilada sauce and bake at 350° F. for approximately 25 minutes.

Easy Bean Quesadillas

I have featured this dish in a class that was designed for cooking for kids.

1 package whole-wheat pita bread (or whole-wheat flour tortillas)

½ onion, chopped fine

1 cup finely chopped green pepper

1 can refried beans (or see Refried Bean recipe on page 135)

¼ cup Monterey Jack Cheese, grated

Salsa

Cook the pita bread or tortillas in saucepan on medium heat until lightly browned and then turn over. (Or you could steam them or bake in a 350° F oven a few minutes.)

In a bowl, combine the onion, green pepper, beans and cheese. If using pita bread, gently split in half. Then spread 1-2 tablespoons of the bean/cheese mixture and close. If using tortillas, fill and cover each of the tortillas with another tortilla. If you like, spray the tops of the tortillas with olive oil vegetable spray. Bake the quesadillas for 5 minutes in a 400° F. oven or until the cheese has melted. Serve with salsa.

This is a recipe that kids can make. Heat the tortillas and place the vegetables, green pepper, cheese and salsa in separate bowls and let them make their own.

Mexican Wrap-Ups

These are a great picnic food. You can make them ahead of time, or put them together when you get there:

1 package corn tortillas

Bean mixture:

2 cups cooked red kidney beans, undrained

Olive oil or olive oil spray

1 onion, chopped

3 stalks celery, chopped

1 16-ounce can crushed tomatoes

2 cloves garlic, minced

4 tablespoons chili powder

Dash of cayenne pepper

1 teaspoon cumin powder or Chili seasoning mix

  (medium)

Condiments: Salsa and chopped onions

Cooking beans from scratch: Wash and rinse beans well. Soak overnight and drain off water. Bring beans to a boil, cover, reduce heat and let them simmer about 2 hours.

Sauté onion and celery in a pan sprayed with olive oil or olive oil spray. Combine the cooked or canned beans with the vegetables and chili seasonings. Bring to a light boil and let simmer 10-15 minutes.

To assemble: Put one or two tablespoons of bean mixture on top of corn tortilla; add salsa and roll up and secure with a toothpick. Serve immediately.

Variation: To make a Vegetarian Chili dish, don't drain the beans. Serve with a side salad.

Mediterranean Rollups

Great for picnics or a Mexican theme dinner.

12 whole-wheat flour tortillas

Filling:

**2 cups cooked garbanzo beans, or 1 can garbanzo
  beans, drained**

2 tablespoons herb wine or brown rice vinegar

¼ teaspoon garlic powder
Salt to taste

½ medium onion, chopped fine

½ teaspoon cumin, coriander, salt and caraway seeds
1 tomato, chopped

1 head green leaf lettuce

1 container alfalfa sprouts or other garden sprouts

**Optional: Mediterranean Humus, Yogurt Cheese Dip,
  or Tofu Dill Dip.**

Combine garbanzos, onions, tomatoes and spices in blender and process until half smooth and still somewhat chunky. In the meantime, heat tortillas until soft and pliable; warm for 30 seconds in a non-stick skillet over medium heat, or in a 350° F. oven for a minute or so. Before assembling, lightly moisten the tortillas, one at a time. Spread ½ cup of the mixture on the tortilla and add some lettuce and sprouts. Roll up into a tight tube. If you want, place four toothpicks along roll. Using a very sharp knife, slice the rolls into approximately one-inch lengths.

Optional: Arrange on a plate or a large platter, leaving room in the center for some Mediterranean Humus, Yogurt Cheese Dip or Tofu Dill Dip.

Dill White Bean Pasta

Here's an easy dish to whip up for dinner. It's colorful and nutritious!

2 cups cooked radiatore, bowtie, corkscrew or rotelli pasta

1 head broccoli, lightly steamed

Dressing:

2 tablespoons olive oil

¼ cup Italian herb wine vinegar or apple cider vinegar

¼ teaspoon salt

1 tablespoon dried dill

2 cups cooked or canned Great Northern white beans, drained

¼ cup black olives, chopped

¼ cup parsley, chopped

Cook pasta according to directions, drain and put aside. Next, steam the broccoli for 4-5 minutes. In the meantime, make the dressing in a separate bowl or blender. Toss the pasta, broccoli, beans, olives, parsley and dressing and then serve.

Bean Burrito

This is another easy recipe that is great for children to make.

2 16-ounce cans red beans, drained (or cooked, see
  bean cooking)
1 small onion, chopped and sautéed
Dash of chili powder and cumin
5-6 whole-wheat or corn tortillas
Salsa or favorite enchilada sauce

Mash beans in a food processor or blender. Add sautéed onion and spices. Meanwhile, heat the tortillas in a pre-heated oven or toaster oven. Place one tablespoon of beans on the tortilla and top with chopped tomatoes and salsa. Roll and serve with a little extra salsa on the side.

(See bean soup and chili section for more bean recipes.)

Chapter Seventeen

Soups and Chilies

Soups are easy to make and are great as a side dish or a simple meal. Almost all vegetables lend themselves to soups: celery, mushrooms, carrots, peas, cabbage, tomatoes, zucchini, cauliflower, red peppers. Generally, add vegetables toward the end of cooking and simmer until they are tender. Vegetables such as garlic and onions can be lightly sautéed at the beginning of the preparation to add flavor.

For heartier soups, try different beans like red, navy, aduki, black, black eyed peas, lentils, split peas and grains such as barley, rice, oats, and millet.

Soups also combine foods such as beans, vegetables, grains, liquid and seasonings. Herbs that lend themselves to soups are ginger, basil, mint, garlic, oregano, fennel, thyme, rosemary and dill.

For light broths, use finely cut vegetables. Thickened soups use beans, pasta and heartier vegetables.

For soup stocks: Simmer leftover vegetables for 10-15 minutes in water and drain. Use the liquid for your base. Season with onion, garlic, bay leaf, thyme and marjoram.

There are many soup broths available on the market. Barth's is one type that is delicious and comes in beef, chicken and vegetable styles. Health Valley also makes a canned chicken broth, available in both low or non-fat styles.

To thicken soups naturally without dairy:

•Puree two cooked potatoes with or without the skins. Add to creamy soups and other sauces.

•Add 1 cup blended silken tofu, which offers the richness and consistency of cream. Good for corn, potato and mushroom soups.

•Add ¼-½ cup oats, oat flour or oat meal. After the soup is cooked, add the oats, oat meal, or oat flour and puree.

•After the soup is cooked, take out half of the soup and blend it in a blender. Add to other half and mix well.

Healthy Vegetable Stock Broth

Here is a recipe for not only a stock broth, but a healthy alkalizing drink:

1 bunch asparagus

1 head broccoli

1-2 onions

1-3 carrots

1-2 zucchinis

Cook chopped vegetables in water. Simmer for 20-30 minutes. Drain vegetables and keep the broth. This is a healthy drink, especially if you are recovering from illness. You can also simmer these vegetables and put them in a blender. This will make a vegetable puree-type soup that is also healthy to drink. You will want to flavor this with some salt and Italian seasonings.

Hearty Vegetable Stew

Here's a nice basic stew recipe, great for cold weather.

2 onions, chopped

2 carrots, chopped

4 stalks celery, chopped

1 potato, peeled and chopped

1 green pepper, chopped

1 cup broccoli crowns, chopped

½ teaspoon salt

½ teaspoon paprika

Dash of cayenne pepper

Dash of cumin

2-3 tablespoons vegetable broth powder

Optional: cooked stew meat

Sauté onions in a saucepan sprayed with olive oil or Pam olive oil pump spray. Stir gently until onions are translucent. Add carrots, celery, potato, green pepper and broccoli, Sauté a few minutes and add spices. Cover with water and bring to a boil. Turn flame to low and simmer 30 minutes.

Alphabet Vegetable Soup

I made this for a children's cooking class, but it's great for adults, too, and simple to make.

1-2 cups cooked Alphabet noodles

Vegetable spray

1 onion, chopped

1 carrot, chopped

1 cup of peas (frozen)

1-2 tomatoes, chopped

2 stalks celery, chopped

1 potato, chopped

Vegetarian soup stock (3 teaspoons in 1 cup liquid)

Salt, or garlic salt to taste

Cook pasta according to directions, drain and put aside. Sauté onion in a pan sprayed with vegetable spray. Then add remaining ingredients. Add water to cover vegetables with vegetarian soup stock. An easy way to make this soup is to use chopped frozen stew vegetables, which normally comes with onions, carrots, celery and potato. Add a chopped tomato and peas. Bring to a boil and simmer for about 20 minutes. Season to taste.

Cream of Tomato Soup

This is great! I substitute tofu for cream in this creamy, hearty tomato soup.

Olive oil

1 onion, minced

1 clove garlic, minced

8 ounces firm tofu, cubed

6 cherry tomatoes, or 3 medium tomatoes, chopped

¾ cups water

5 mushrooms, chopped

1 teaspoon cumin

2 tablespoons soy sauce

Sauté onions and garlic in olive oil until they are translucent. Add water, tomatoes, mushrooms, tofu, and spices. Cool. Pour in a food processor or blender and process until smooth. Serve hot or cold. Sprinkle with parsley. **Optional:** add remaining tofu cubes. **Variations:** ½ teaspoon each: cumin, oregano, thyme, marjoram and basil.

French Onion Soup

A great vegetarian version of a traditional soup. Use a broth powder, or if desired, flavor with a mild miso paste. If you like the taste of miso, you could replace the Tamari soy sauce with 3-4 tablespoons of brown rice miso. The classes all surprised me with wanting to try brown rice miso in this soup, and they loved it! Otherwise, just use the recipe as follows.

3-4 tablespoons of beef or chicken vegetable broth powder in 1 cup water

2-3 cloves garlic, minced

3 onions, sliced finely

2 teaspoons olive oil (optional)

3-4 tablespoons soy sauce (or 1 tablespoon miso)

Parmesan Cheese

Croutons:

6-8 slices whole-wheat toast

Vegetable spray

1 garlic clove

Sauté onion and garlic in a saucepan lightly sprayed with vegetable oil. Add vegetable broth, cover and cook 25 minutes. Garnish with scallions and parsley.

Easy healthy croutons: Rub both sides of bread with garlic and brush with olive oil or vegetable spray. Toast the bread or put in a 350° F oven for a few minutes. Take out when toasted, and carefully cut three times lengthwise and then crosswise three times with a serrated knife. To serve, pour bowl of soup. Sprinkle croutons and some Parmesan cheese on top of soup.

Minestrone

A real hit! I like using the Muir Glenn brand of tomato paste. This soup is spicy, thick and delicious.

2 cups cooked Great Northern beans or white kidney beans, undrained

Vegetable spray

2 cloves garlic, minced

1 onion, peeled and chopped

2 carrots, chopped fine

2 celery stalks, chopped fine

3 tomatoes, chopped

2 potatoes, chopped

1 cup vegetable stock (2-3 tablespoons Barth's broth powder diluted in 1 cup water)

1 teaspoon oregano

¼ teaspoon basil

½ teaspoon salt

Dash cayenne pepper, to taste

1 cup uncooked pasta (tiny shells)

1 small can of tomato paste

Sauté onion and garlic in a pan sprayed with vegetable spray. Add carrots, celery, tomatoes and potatoes. Add water to cover (about 4-6 cups) and simmer vegetables for about 10 minutes. Add beans and spices. Bring to a boil and add the uncooked pasta. Simmer for 10-15 minutes more until the pasta is done.

Note: An easy way to put this soup together is to simply substitute a package of frozen stew vegetables for the fresh ones which normally contains onion, carrots, celery and potatoes. Then just add a chopped tomato.

Cuban Black Bean Soup

*This is a great rendition of a traditional soup. I've exper-
imented and found that just a teaspoon of the vinegar really
makes this soup. Well liked by everyone.*

1 cup dry black beans or

2 cups cooked black beans (1-2 cans, undrained)

1-2 tablespoons Barth's or broth powder

2 bay leaves

6 cups water

1 onion, chopped fine

1 green pepper, chopped

2 cloves garlic, minced

½ teaspoon oregano, cumin and basil

½ teaspoon salt

1 teaspoon white wine vinegar or lemon juice

Dash of cayenne and paprika

If using dry beans, sort beans, wash well and rinse. Soak
overnight in water. Discard water. Bring 6 cups of water to
a boil with bay leaves. Reduce heat to low and let simmer for
2 hours or until tender. If you want to use canned beans, omit
this step.

Meanwhile, sauté onion, green peppers, and garlic. Add
cooked or canned beans with the other spices and simmer for
about 15-20 minutes. When the beans are tender, serve as
they are, or remove half of the beans and puree them in a
blender. Then pour them back in the pot with the soup and
serve.

Variation: To make a sweeter soup, add 1 teaspoon
honey.

Creamy Blackbean and Pumpkin Stew

This is easy to make and delicious.

1 onion, chopped

1 can pumpkin puree

2 tablespoons vegetable broth powder diluted in 1 cup
water

1 can black beans, undrained

2 cups milk (or soy milk, water or 1 cup blended tofu)

1 teaspoon salt

1 teaspoon basil

1 tablespoon soy sauce to taste

Garnish: toasted pumpkin seeds

Sauté onion in a saucepan sprayed with vegetable spray.
Combine pumpkin puree, broth, beans water and seasonings.
Bring to a boil, and simmer for 10-15 minutes. Serve with
toasted pepitas or pumpkin seeds on top. Serve in a hallowed
-out pumpkin or mini pumpkin.

Pasta E Fagiole

2 cups wheat or Jerusalem artichoke pasta shells,
cooked

1 clove garlic, minced

1 small onion, minced

1 15-ounce can chopped or crushed tomatoes

1 tablespoon Italian seasoning

1 16-ounce can white beans, drained

2 cups vegetable stock

½ teaspoon each: basil, salt and white pepper

Cook pasta according to instructions on package.
Meanwhile, sauté onion, garlic and then add Italian seasoning
and canned tomatoes. Bring to medium high heat and simmer

for 10 minutes. Add beans and vegetable stock to the pot and simmer for 20 minutes. Drain pasta, add and simmer for 3 minutes. Serve with a side Italian or Greek salad and whole-grain bread.

Chilies

Chili, corn bread and a salad makes a great healthy meal. Chili can be made with many beans: black, pinto, kidney, lentils or aduki, or even white beans. Chilies can be made even quicker using a commercial chili mix like The Spice Hunter Chili Mix, an all-natural, no-salt mix which combines chili, onion, garlic, cocoa powder, oregano, cayenne, cumin, cinnamon and cloves.

Vegetarian Chili

A great hit! Even husbands like this dish. The tempeh adds a real meat-like flavor and texture.

1½ cups chopped onion

1 cup chopped green, yellow and red peppers

2 14½-ounce can chopped or crushed tomatoes

2 16-ounce cans kidney beans, undrained

2½ tablespoons chili powder

1½ teaspoons ground cumin

1 teaspoon dried oregano

¼ teaspoon white pepper

½ teaspoon salt
2 tablespoons minced garlic or garlic powder

Dash of cayenne pepper

Optional: 8 ounces tempeh, grated, seasoned with

  2-3 tablespoons of soy sauce or Tamari

1 can tomato paste (makes a more sweeter chili)

Sauté onion first. Then if using tempeh, add grated tempeh seasoned with soy sauce and sauté a few minutes. Add the peppers and sauté. Add the crushed tomatoes, kidney beans and spices. Bring to a boil, cover and reduce heat and simmer 20 minutes, stirring occasionally.

Red Bean Chili ✒

Another great chili dish

2 cups red kidney beans, dried

6 cups water

or 2 cans kidney beans, not drained

1 onion, chopped

3 stalks celery, chopped

1 16-ounce can crushed tomatoes

2 cloves garlic, minced

1 can tomato sauce

4 tablespoons chili powder

Dash of cayenne pepper

1 teaspoon cumin powder

If cooking beans from scratch, wash and rinse beans well. Soak overnight and drain off water. Bring beans to a boil, cover, reduce heat and let them simmer about 2 hours. Meanwhile, sauté onion and celery in a pan sprayed with vegetable spray. Combine the beans with the onion/celery mix and add the rest of the ingredients. Let simmer another 2 hours.

If using canned beans, combine undrained beans with the remaining ingredients and let simmer on low for about 1 hour.

White Bean Chili

This is tasty and was a great hit, too. Use white beans and green chilis for spice.

3 cups water

1½ cups Great Northern beans

or 1 can Great Northern beans

2 leeks, chopped

1 yellow pepper, chopped

1 large onion, chopped

2 cloves garlic, minced

2 stalks celery

½ teaspoon cumin

3 teaspoons vegetarian chicken broth in ¼ cup water

1 can Green Enchilada Sauce (or 1 can green chilies, drained)

¼ teaspoon cayenne

1 teaspoon salt

If cooking beans from scratch, soak 1 cup Great Northern beans in 3 cups water for 8 hours. Pour off water. Put beans in pot and cover with water and cook 1-1 1/2 hours. During the last half hour, add spices. If cooking beans from scratch, the chicken broth is optional.

If using canned beans, you will add them after you cook the vegetables. Sauté onion, garlic and leeks. Add the remaining vegetables and spices. Cook with low heat for 30 minutes. Add one can of drained beans and continue to cook until beans are thoroughly heated, but not mushy.

Simple Chili

Quick, low-fat and delicious!

1 cup pinto beans, cooked

2 cloves garlic, minced

1 can tomatoes, crushed

2 tablespoons chili powder

Add spices and tomatoes to cooked beans. Cover and then simmer for 30 minutes.

Chapter Eighteen

Tofu and Tempeh

Soybeans are an added boost to almost any diet. High in protein, and low in fat, they contain no cholesterol. They do contain a type of natural estrogen which has been most helpful for women going through menopause.

Tofu

Tofu is a convenient nutritious food which can take on any flavor, from spicy to sweet. Tofu is simply a food made from soybeans. Soybeans are cooked, blended, and then curdled with a curdling agent such as Nigari, and poured through a cotton sieve into a square box. This is a process similar to produce cheese curds from animal milk. In Asia tofu is sometimes called "meat of the fields" or "soy cheese."

There are many forms of tofu available: silken or soft, firm and extra firm. Silken tofu blends the best and mixes more thoroughly than regular tofu. Soft tofu is suited for creamy dressings, dips and dessert recipes such as pudding or pie fillings (See Easy and Quick Tofu Chocolate Pudding on page 216). Firm and extra firm are the most versatile. Firm tofu is best for recipes that call for slicing or dicing. Tofu can be mashed, blended, crumbled or sliced. Tofu is low in calories. There are only 164 calories in 8 ounces. It's also rich in organic calcium. There is the same amount of calcium in 8 ounces of tofu as there is in 8 ounces of milk.

Tofu is high in iron. Eight ounces of tofu supplies the same amount of iron as 2 ounces of beef liver or 4 eggs.

Tofu has high-quality protein. Eight ounces supplies the same amount of protein as 2 eggs, 2 ounces of regular cheese, 1 ½ cup milk, or 5½ ounces of hamburger, and best of all, tofu is lower in fat than any of these.

Other uses for Tofu: Tofu can be used in spaghetti, chili, stir fries, salads, scrambled, sweet and sour, salad dressings, dips, spreads, beverages, drinks and desserts. Tofu also can be purchased pre-cooked or marinated and eaten as a delicious snack. There are commercial tofu burgers and tofu hot dogs available in most health food stores.

Ways to Use Tofu

1. Use tofu as a meat substitute. Combine a half pound of crumbled tofu with a half pound of ground meat for making hamburgers, meatballs, meat loaf or foods such as stuffed green peppers or cabbage. Or substitute tofu chunks for some or all the meat in stews.

2. Substitute crumbled tofu for hamburger meat in tacos. Top with usual chopped tomato, cheese, and onions.

3. Dice tofu in quarter-inch cubes and combine with eggs for scrambling. Or combine tofu with eggs for egg salad.

4. Use tofu to make your soups creamy without using cream. Add the tofu to the soup and blend. Serve hot or cold.

5. Use crumbled tofu as a substitute for part or all the ricotta cheese when making lasagna.

6. Make a peanut butter spread with a half-pound of tofu and a half cup of peanut butter. Add raisins or sunflower seeds.

7. Store tofu in the refrigerator immersed with water. Change the water every other day. Tofu can stay fresh up to two weeks.

8. Always drain tofu before using, especially if using soft tofu.

Tofu Quiche

This is great! If you miss the taste of quiche made with eggs, you'll want to try this quiche. The tofu has the texture like eggs, without the added dairy.

Filling:

16 ounces firm Tofu, (grated)

¼ cup cold-pressed olive oil

2 cups sliced, sautéed mushrooms

1 medium onion, chopped fine

1-6 ounce package frozen spinach

2 cloves garlic, minced

¼ cup soy sauce

½ teaspoon blackstrap molasses

Whole-wheat pie crust:

1 cup whole-wheat pastry flour

½ teaspoon salt

¼ cup olive oil or Spectrum Spread

6 tablespoons cold water

Preheat oven to 350° F.

Filling: Cut tofu in half and put half in blender and blend until smooth. Lay aside.

In a sauce pan, sauté onions and garlic and add the mushrooms, soy sauce and blackstrap molasses. Simmer until onions are soft. Grate the other half of tofu and combine with the garlic onion mixture.

Crust: To make the pie crust, combine the flour and salt. Beat the oil and ice water together with a wire whisk until thick. Pour the oil and water mixture over the flour and salt, mixing until all the flour is moistened. If too dry, add more water, just a little at a time. Roll out the dough on floured surface, or between two layers of waxed paper. Put pie crust in a pie plate and bake for 10 minutes at 375° F before filling. Then spoon the tofu mixture into the partially-baked whole-wheat pie crust. Bake at 350° F. for 25 to 30 minutes. Let stand 5-10 minutes before cutting.

Hawaiian Vegetables with Tofu

Yum, Yum! Another classic hit.

Olive oil vegetable spray

1 small onion, sliced in crescent moon shapes

½ red, green, yellow pepper, diagonally sliced

1 8-ounce can water chestnuts, chopped

1 15-ounce can unsweetened pineapple chunks, drained but keep juice

1 8-ounce carton tofu

2 tablespoons soy sauce

2 tablespoons cornstarch powder

¼ cup brown rice vinegar

¼ cup honey

½-¾ cup pineapple juice

½ teaspoon garlic powder

1 teaspoon dried ginger root

Optional: ¼ cup slivered almonds

Chow Mein noodles or cooked brown rice

Sauté the onion in a small saucepan sprayed with vegetable spray until onions are translucent. Add peppers, water chestnuts, pineapple and tofu. In a bowl, combine the soy sauce, cornstarch powder, vinegar, honey, pineapple juice and spices together. Add to the tofu mixture and cook over medium heat until mixture starts to boil. Serve over cooked noodles or brown rice.

Tofu Stir-fry

An easy way to cook tofu. You may want to marinate tofu first in a marinade of ¼ cup Tamari soy sauce and ¼ cup brown rice vineger. Then use in sauté.

Pam spray

One cabbage, shredded

3 carrots, grated

½ teaspoon dillweed

½ teaspoon tarragon

2 teaspoons lemon juice

½ teaspoon salt

1 block tofu, cut in cubes

Lightly coat saucepan with Pam spray. Add cabbage, carrots and stir. Sauté four minutes. Add spices and toss. Add tofu and continue sautéeing for 4 more minutes. Toss with lemon and serve.

Tofu Cheese Scramble

Here is a great breakfast for people who don't eat eggs.

1 pound firm tofu, crumbled

¼ teaspoon salt

Dash of white pepper

½ cup grated Mozzarella cheese

¼ Feta cheese, crumbled

In skillet, heat olive oil over medium-high heat. Add tofu, spices and sauté until heated, stirring. Add cheese and cook until melted. Serve hot.

Mushroom Stroganoff

The tofu is used here as a substitute for cream. Use as much as you need to attain the desired results. The flavors are great!

Olive oil vegetable spray

1½ cup onions, chopped

3 cloves garlic, minced

1 teaspoon dillweed

2 teaspoons basil

1-2 teaspoons soy sauce (or Bragg's Amino Acids)

4-5 cups mushrooms, chopped

½ teaspoon salt

¼ teaspoon cayenne

2 16-ounces firm tofu, blended

2 teaspoons dried parsley

1 package orzo pasta or brown rice

Spray a saucepan with a light coat of olive oil spray. Quickly sauté onions, garlic and spices. Add soy sauce, mushrooms, salt and cayenne. Cook 5 minutes over lower heat.   Add tofu and parsley to mushroom mixture and combine well.   Cook pasta or brown rice. Pour stroganoff over pasta or brown rice and serve.

Tempeh

Tempeh (tem-pay) has been a staple in Indonesia for thousands of years. A combination of soybeans and grains which are fermented together, it's a good source of healthy bacteria that keeps the colon healthy. Tempeh is very high in protein (16 grams per 1/3 of a block), and contains other beneficial vitamins and minerals found in soybeans and grains. It also contains 6 grams of fiber and 5 grams of fat. White Wave Tempeh comes in several varieties: sea veggie, soy rice, soy, wild rice and five grain (millet, oats, barley, wheat, brown rice), and needs to be steamed, baked or sautéed before eating.

Tempeh is also versatile. I like to grate it and sauté it with onions, garlic and vegetables and then use in place of meat in many recipes: spaghetti, chili, vegetarian egg rolls, and lasagne.

Mock Tuna Salad Filling

Many people have been surprised with how much tempeh can be like tuna salad in this salad. Tempeh has a nice chunky texture and like tofu, takes on the flavorings that are combined with it. This is a great, low-fat, low cholesterol salad.

1 package of tempeh, steamed

½ cup onions, green onions or leeks, chopped fine

2 stalks celery, shopped fine

3 tablespoons Dijon mustard

¼ cup mayonnaise (I like Nayonaise or Lite Canola Mayonnaise)

Salt, white pepper to taste

1 clove garlic or dash garlic powder

3 pieces whole-wheat bread

Optional: 1 head leaf lettuce

162

Steam tempeh in steamer or lightly simmer in water for 20 minutes. Let cool and mash with a potato masher or your hands. Combine the vegetables with the mustard, mayonnaise and spices and use as a filling for whole-wheat sandwiches: Place a couple tablespoons of mock tuna salad on one slice of bread. Cover with another slice of wheat bread and spread another layer of mock tuna salad. Cover with another slice of bread and cut into fourths, securing each one with a toothpick.

Hungarian Goulash

Another dish that was well liked in the cooking classes.

Vegetable spray

1 medium onion, chopped

2 cloves garlic, minced

8 ounces tempeh, grated or chopped fine

2 tablespoons soy sauce (or Bragg's Amino Acids)

4 tomatoes, chopped

2 stalks celery, chopped

8 mushrooms, chopped

½-1 teaspoon salt (or salt to taste)

½-1 teaspoon white pepper (or to taste)

3 tablespoons ground paprika

2 tablespoons whole-wheat pastry flour

Dash of cayenne pepper

Optional: 1 can tomato paste

1 package kamut macaroni noodles (or quinoa, whole-wheat or brown rice elbow macaroni noodles, or quinoa wheat-free veggie curls)

Sauté onion and garlic in a saucepan coated with vegetable spray. Add tempeh and Tamari and continue to cook. Add tomatoes, celery, mushrooms, and spices and cook until spices blend. Do not boil. Serve over or stir in hot cooked macaroni. Have soy sauce on hand for further seasoning.

I've made this same dish with red beans. You could add 2 cans of drained pinto or red beans in place of, or in addition to the tempeh. Or, you could use Ready Ground Tofu in place of the tempeh. (Use only half of the package and add like you would the beans.) The Ancient Harvest quinoa wheat-free veggie curls are delicious. Cleopatra's Kamut pasta has the orzo and macaroni elbow styles.

Vegetable Paella

This traditional Spanish dish is great, and even better with natural herbs and spices.

1 cup of dry brown rice (or 2 cups cooked)

5 cloves garlic, minced

1 onion, chopped

1 green or yellow pepper, chopped

1 red pepper, chopped

2 tablespoons walnuts or almonds, chopped

3 tomatoes, chopped

1 cup green peas

1 teaspoon cumin

¼ teaspoon turmeric

Dash of cayenne pepper

1 cup water

1 package tempeh, thawed

Optional: Grated Parmesan cheese

Option 1: If cooking brown rice, wash 1 cup brown rice, drain and add 2 cups water. Bring to a boil and simmer 55-60 minutes. Follow rest of recipe except omit the cup of water.

Option 2: If using uncooked brown rice, sauté onion and garlic in lightly oiled saucepan. Cut the tempeh into small chunks. Add washed and drained brown rice, tempeh, water and rest of ingredients. Reduce heat to low and simmer 1 hour. Grated soy cheese is optional.

Vegetarian Egg Rolls

These were a real hit. You can use turkey or chicken meat instead of tempeh, using the same spices.

Filling:

1 8-ounces package tempeh, thawed and grated

1 onion, minced

1 clove garlic, minced

¼ teaspoon ginger root

1 cup finely shredded cabbage

½ cup shredded carrots

1 can bamboo shoots, drained and diced

3 tablespoons soy sauce or Bragg's Amino Acids

1 tablespoon cornstarch or arrowroot powder diluted in ¼ -½ cup water

Salt to taste

Optional: ¼ cup crushed cashews

1 package egg roll wrappers (Naysoya)

Sealer mixture: 1 teaspoon flour; 1 tablespoon water

  Optional: egg whites

Egg rolls may sound difficult, but they are actually easy to put together. Commercially pre-made wrappers are available at most oriental grocery stores.

To make filling: Cut up fine or grate 1 package of tempeh. Set aside. Sauté onion, garlic, ginger root and grated tempeh in a sauce pan sprayed with olive oil vegetable spray. Add cabbage, carrots and bamboo shoots. Combine diluted cornstarch and soy sauce and stir well. Add this to the vegetable mixture and stir one minute.

Sealer mix: in a small bowl, mix 1 teaspoon flour and 1 tablespoon water.

To assemble: Place 2 tablespoon of filling diagonally across one wrapper. Fold like a baby's diaper: the first fold the bottom corner over filling, and then fold the left and right corners. Roll up the egg roll to enclose the filling. Then seal the filling with a sealer mix.

To bake, place them on a cookie sheet that has been lightly sprayed with vegetable spray. Then lightly spray the egg rolls with vegetable spray so they don't dry out. (Or you could "wash" with an egg white). Bake for 10-15 minutes in a 400° F preheated oven. After they are lightly browned on top, gently turn them over and bake 10 more minutes. Serve with a mustard or sweet and sour sauce.

Mustard sauce: 2 tablespoons Dijon mustard, 1 teaspoon honey, 1 teaspoon brown rice vinegar

Sweet and sour sauce: 3 tablespoons apple sauce, 3 tablespoons apple cider vinegar, 1 tablespoon honey, 1 teaspoon ginger root powder.

Stuffed Green Peppers

Here's a delicious alternative to meat stuffings:

4-5 green peppers, halved and seeded

Stuffing:

1 package five-grain tempeh, grated

1½ teaspoon Worcestershire sauce

½ teaspoon salt

¼ teaspoon white pepper

¼ **teaspoon garlic powder**

1 teaspoon dried parsley

1 cup of corn kernels (canned, fresh or frozen)

1 cup of green peas (canned, fresh or frozen)

¾ **cup whole-wheat bread crumbs (I like Jaclyn's)**

¼ **cup barbecue sauce (I like Enricos)**

2-4 tablespoons of water as necessary

Optional: Mozzarella cheese

Carefully remove tops from peppers, take out seeds, and slice peppers in half. Put in a steamer and steam for about 5-8 minutes, until they still retain their green color. Set aside.

In the meantime, sauté onion in a pan sprayed with vegetable spray and add grated tempeh. Add spices and continue to sauté until tempeh is well flavored. Add corn, green peas, bread crumbs and barbecue sauce and mix well. Add water if necessary. Heat through. Fill each pepper with mixture. Since the peppers were steamed and the tempeh has been cooked, you don't have to bake this dish any more. Place peppers on a serving dish. If you like, top with a small amount of shredded Mozzarella cheese. (You can put in a 350° F. oven for 5 minutes to let the cheese melt.)

Tempeh Reuben Sandwiches on Rye

I loved eating Reuben sandwiches when I was growing up, but I stopped eating them because of their high-fat content. This recipe is a great alternative to those tasty sandwiches which are usually high-fat. Cascadian Farms makes the best sauerkraut I've ever eaten. Naysoya makes a tofu-based Thousand Island dressing that is just like the original high-fat dressing. The cheese is optional: a low-fat Swiss is nice. TofuRella makes a nice Garlic Herb Cheese Dressing that works well too. And in the classes, people chose between Thousand Island dressing or mustard.

8 ounces tempeh

1-2 ounces shredded Swiss Cheese

1-2 ounces Sauerkraut

3 pieces rye bread

**Dressings: Thousand Island Dressing (I like Nasoya)
     or mustard**

Steam tempeh for 20 minutes. Slice tempeh in half and then cut each half into 2-3 pieces. To make sandwiches: On a slice of sauerkraut rye bread, place a slice of tempeh and cover with sauerkraut and grated Swiss cheese. Place a piece of rye bread on top and repeat layer of tempeh, cheese and sauerkraut. Top with one more piece of rye bread. Place under a broiler for 1-2 minutes to melt the cheese and brown the bread. Remove and turn upside down and broil 1-2 more minutes. Take out and open the sandwich to add the dressing. Cut the sandwich into four pieces using a sharp knife. Secure each piece with a toothpick and serve warm.

Easy Sloppy Joes

I grew up ejoying Sloppy Joes for lunch. Mom made this dish with hamburger meat. It was a quick meal and we all really loved it. Here's my version made with tempeh.

1 package tempeh, grated

1 onion, chopped fine

1-2 teaspoons olive oil

Hearty Spaghetti Sauce (page 103)

Sauté tempeh and onions in 1-2 teaspoons of olive oil. Add Hearty Spaghetti Sauce and simmer 15 minutes. Serve over whole-grain bread and accompany with a side green salad. Sprinkle Paramesan cheese on top.

Tempeh Loaf and Easy Gravy

Here is a great vegetarian type of meat loaf that could be served for a special occasion with the Easy Gravy recipe (page 106.) I did this for a Thanksgiving cooking class I taught, along with the gravy recipe, Cranberry Sauce, Mashed Sweet Potatoes, Classic Salad, and Pumpkin Pie. Everyone rated the dishes very high.

Vegetable spray

1 onion, chopped fine

16 ounces tempeh, grated

2 tablespoons vegetable powder (diluted in 1 cup water)

2 cups whole-wheat bread crumbs

1 tablespoon soy sauce or ½ teaspoon sea salt

½ teaspoon oregano

½ teaspoon thyme

½ teaspoon basil

Grate tempeh with a grater. Sauté onion in vegetable spray and add tempeh. Sauté 5 minutes. Add the rest of the ingredients and mix well. Pack mixture in a oiled bread loaf pan. Cover with foil and bake at 350° F, for 30 minutes. Serve with Easy Gravy recipe found on page 106.

Chapter Nineteen

Winning Ways With Chicken

Chicken is perhaps the most versatile meat available. You can do more with chicken than other meats because of its nice flavor. Chicken combines well with vegetables, grains, eggs, and tomatoes. I prefer to buy "free-range" chicken meat which means the chickens have been allowed to range, rather than be cooped up in small pens. Free-range chickens are healthier and leaner, and are usually fed healthier foods.

Most people have a zillion recipes for chicken already. I've made some of the more familiar recipes with more natural, healthy ingredients.

Curried Chicken and Vegetables

This will add a bit of spice to your life!

1 chicken breast, skinned and bones and sliced

1 teaspoon olive oil

¼ cup chopped scallions
1 clove garlic, minced

1 cup each: mushrooms and green peppers, chopped

½ cup chopped tomatoes
1 teaspoon lemon juice

1 teaspoon salt

2 tablespoons curry powder

Sauté scallions and garlic in olive oil in a saucepan. Add vegetables and stir-fry for a few minutes. Transfer to a dish and sauté the sliced chicken in olive oil. stir-fry 4 minutes. Add the vegetables to the chicken, then add the lemon juice, spices and stir well. You can serve this over brown rice or whole-grain noodles.

Chicken Cheese Enchilada

These are great, easy to fix and delicious, too. Another hit in the cooking classes.

8-10 corn or flour tortillas

Olive oil or olive oil spray

2 cups chicken strips, cut up

1 cup low-fat Mozzarella cheese, grated (optional)

Enchilada Sauce:

1 small can tomato paste

4-5 teaspoons chili powder

¼ teaspoon each: oregano, cumin, garlic and onion powder

2 cups water (or more as needed)

2 tablespoons corn meal

Combine together in a saucepan and cook for 10 minutes.

To assemble enchiladas: Spray a 9 x 13-inch baking dish with olive oil mist spray. First, lightly dip tortillas one at a time in the sauce and fill each with some chicken strips and grated Mozzarella cheese. Roll up and place in baking dish, next to each other. Continue to fill each one until the filling and tortillas are used. Cover with Enchilada Sauce and bake at 350° F. for approximately 25 minutes.

Chicken Cacciatore

A quick, tasty, fairly low-fat recipe.

4 boneless chicken breasts

1 tablespoon olive oil or spray

1 cup onions, chopped

1 cup mushrooms, chopped

1 cup green peppers, chopped

2 cups tomato puree (no sugar, low salt)

¼ teaspoon white pepper
l clove garlic

1 teaspoon each oregano and paprika

Sauté chicken breasts in Pam or oil until brown. Put aside. Sauté onion, mushrooms, green peppers and spices. Add tomato puree and bring to a boil and stir until thick. Add chicken and simmer together 5 minutes. Spoon sauce over chicken when you serve it.

Chicken Ratatouille

1 medium eggplant, cubed

1 onion, chopped

2 cloves garlic, minced

1 each red and green pepper, chopped

1 8-ounce can tomatoes

1 pound chicken breast cut into strips

Olive oil

Sauté garlic and onions with small amount of oil. Add remaining ingredients and simmer 30 minutes, turning chicken halfway through.

Chicken Oriental Stir-fry

If you're tired of grilled chicken, here's a nice variation.

2 large chicken breasts, cut in strips

½ head Chinese cabbage or Savoy cabbage

4 stalks celery, sliced diagonally

4 green onions, chopped diagonally

1 stalk broccoli, chopped

1 cup of pea pods

1 stalk broccoli, chopped

1 8-ounce can sliced water chestnuts

1-2 carrots, slice on slant

2 cloves garlic, minced

¼ cup water

¼ cup soy sauce

3 teaspoons cornstarch or arrowroot powder

Slowly heat 1 tablespoon canola oil in a wok and brown chicken strips. Sauté garlic and onions. Add all the vegetables except for sprouts and cook quickly until tender, over lower heat. Add remaining vegetables and continue to cook. Separately mix together corn starch or arrowroot powder and ¼ cup water. Then add to vegetables and stir over low heat. Add soy sauce and serve.

Herbed Chicken

Another delicious variation for chicken.

½ pound boneless chicken

2 tablespoons frozen orange juice concentrate

1 teaspoon oregano

¼ teaspoon parsley
1 teaspoon basil

½ teaspoon lemon juice

¼ teaspoon mustard

Preheat broiler and broil chicken. Mix ingredients in a bowl and brush half the mixture over chicken. Broil 10 minutes or until chicken is browned. Base with remaining mixture. Broil 10 minutes longer.

Optional: Add 1 tablespoon lemon juice, ½ teaspoon garlic, or 1 teaspoon Dijon mustard.

Chicken Italian Style

A delicious meal in one pan. Serve with a slice of whole-grain bread.

2 whole chicken breasts, boned and skinned

1 tablespoon olive oil

2 cloves garlic, chopped

½ pound sliced mushrooms
1 medium onion, chopped

2 red or green peppers, chopped

4-5 tomatoes, chopped

¼ teaspoon each parsley, oregano, thyme, marjoram

Brown chicken in oil; add garlic and mushrooms and onions and sauté till tender. Add peppers, tomatoes and spices and cook on low for 3 minutes. You can add cornstarch or arrowroot powder dissolved in ½ cup water to thicken. Let mixture simmer 20 minutes. You can add salt or soy sauce for flavor.

Chicken Parmesan

This was a great hit at Michelle's dinner party. I've cut the Parmesan cheese considerably from the traditional recipe so you still have the flavor and less fat.

4 chicken breasts or 8 sliced thin chicken strips

½ cup Parmesan cheese, grated

1 clove garlic or 1 teaspoon garlic salt

Sauce:

Remaining Parmesan cheese

3-4 tablespoons flour

2 cups chicken stock

1 teaspoon thyme

1 teaspoon tarragon

Optional: Serve over cooked pasta or brown rice

Preheat oven to 350° F. Coat chicken breasts in the cheese and garlic mixture. Place the chicken in a large baking pan which has been sprayed with vegetable olive oil spray. Make the sauce by combining the rest of the Parmesan cheese, chicken stock, flour and spices. Heat in a small saucepan until thick. Pour sauce over chicken and bake for 45 minutes.

Chicken Fajitas

Marinade

2 cloves garlic

2 teaspoons olive oil

6 boneless, skinless chicken breast, cut into ½"
 strips

4 large whole-wheat flour tortillas

Toppings:

1 cup salsa

1 cup non-fat yogurt or sour cream

½ cup mashed avocado

Marinade the chicken for a couple hours in the olive/garlic mixture. Heat a fry pan and sauté chicken strips for about 5-7 minutes in a small amount of olive oil. Meanwhile, wrap the tortillas in aluminum foil and place in a 350° F degree oven. When the chicken is done, remove from heat. To serve, place the chicken in the tortilla. Top with avocado, salsa and yogurt. Roll up and eat.

Chicken Terriyaki

Carol, one of my clients tried this recipe on her family and they loved it. It's spicy and delicious.

6 chicken strips

Marinade:

2 tablespoons soy sauce

1 tablespoon Dijon mustard

2 tablespoons ginger root

2 cloves garlic

1 teaspoon sesame oil

2 cups mushrooms sliced

1 cup green peas

Blend marinade ingredients and pour over chicken. Marinate 1 hour. Place in a wok and stir-fry chicken with a little bit of sesame seed oil. Add vegetables and heat. Serve with rice.

Chicken Chow Mein

1 cup celery, sliced on diagonal

1 medium onion, chopped

1 red pepper, seeded, and cut into strips

1 teaspoon olive oil

1 cup small mushrooms, sliced

1 8-ounce can water chestnuts, rinse and drain

2 tablespoons soy sauce

¾ pound cooked chicken breasts
cooked brown rice and noodles

In olive oil, sauté onions, then celery, pepper, mushrooms and water chestnuts. Add chicken and combine well. Serve over brown rice and sprinkle a few chow mein noodles on top.

Easy Chicken a La King

1 cup cooked chicken

½ cup mushrooms
White Sauce (See recipe on page 107)

When the sauce is smooth, add the chicken and mushrooms. Reduce heat. Serve the chicken as a side dish with vegetables or a salad.

Chapter Twenty

Fabulous Fish and Meat

Animal proteins like fish are very nourishing to our adrenals because they are so rich in protein, and fairly low in calories. Cod has only 109 calories per 4 ounces and whitefish has 175 calories per 4 ounces. Some fish are high in Omega 3 fatty acids. These fish oils can be beneficial for: weight loss, to lower cholesterol, prevent heart disease, build the immune system, prevent cancer, help diabetics, for PMS, skin, nails and candida. They also help lower blood pressure, lower blood cholesterol and to prevent a heart attack.

Fish can be steamed, baked, poached or microwaved with spices and vegetables such as tomatoes, onion, basil, parsley, lemon and olive oil. Experts recommend 3 servings of fish high in Omega 3 oils per week. Fish that are highest in Omega 3 fats are: Mackerel, anchovies, salmon, whitefish and tuna. Cod, perch and trout also contain lower amounts. I recommend cold-water fish and fresh-water fish rather than scavengers such as shrimp, lobster and oysters, which tend to be high in saturated fat. The colder the water, the more benefits of fish oil.) Here are seasoning suggestions.

For halibut: tomatoes, garlic, onion

lemon, thyme, garlic, and vinegar

For baked white fish: cayenne, coriander, garlic,

lemon juice, mustard, white pepper, Dijon mustard,

paprika, and parsley

For red snapper: fennel, bay leaf, lemon, and onions

Dijon Perch

A wonderful flavorful way to prepare perch.

4 perch fillets

¼ cup Dijon mustard

2 tablespoons lemon juice

2 tablespoons water

1 teaspoon white pepper

1 teaspoon thyme

2 tomatoes, chopped

Rinse fish with cold water and pat dry with a paper towel. Place fish on a baking sheet and sprinkle with white pepper. Combine mustard, water, thyme, and tomatoes well and pour over fish. Seal with aluminum foil. Bake at 450° F. for 15-20 minutes or until fish flakes easily when tested. Remove from foil and serve.

Easy Baked or Grilled Fish

An easy way to prepare most light fish.

4 4-ounce cod or whitefish fillets

2 tablespoons Spectrum olive oil

Dash of salt

Dash of cayenne pepper

1 tablespoon minced parsley

¼ cup green onion, minced

2 cloves garlic, minced

2 tablespoons lemon juice

Preheat oven to 400° F. Spray baking pan with olive oil spray or brush with olive oil and place fish. Mix remaining ingredients in a bowl and pour over fish mixture. Bake for 15-20 minutes until fish is flaky.

Easy Salmon Bake

An easy way to use canned or fresh fish.

1 4-ounce can of Salmon (or tuna)

2 tablespoons of olive oil

Salt to taste

Dash of cayenne pepper

¼ cup green onion, minced

2 cloves garlic, minced

2 tablespoons lemon juice

Mix ingredients together and put into a baking dish. Bake at 350° F. for 15 minutes.

Lemon Baked Halibut

You can use this recipe for any light fish.

5 Halibut fillets

1 tablespoons finely minced garlic

1 tablespoons lemon juice

½ teaspoons salt

Sprinkle garlic, lemon juice, and salt over halibut and bake in an oiled. covered pan for 20 minutes in a 350° F. oven.

Marinated Sautéed Salmon Steaks

This was a great hit at a dinner party at Michelle's. You can broil it if you don't want to sauté.

4 4-ounce salmon steaks

Marinade:

4 tablespoons low-sodium soy sauce *liquid aminos*

1 teaspoon fructose, sugar or honey

2 tablespoons olive oil

1½ teaspoons garlic salt or 2 cloves garlic

1 teaspoon dried ginger or 2 tablespoons grated

  ginger root

Mix marinade and marinate salmon for about 15 minutes in the refrigerator. In a large fry pan, over medium high heat, heat one tablespoon of olive oil and gently sauté the salmon steaks for about 4 minutes on each side. Add a sprig of parsley and slice of lemon to garnish.

Low-Fat Healthy Tuna Casserole

One of the few casseroles in this cookbook, this is tasty and even fish eaters enjoy it. It's especially good with a dash of cayenne pepper. Serve with a green salad.

2 cups dry spinach noodles

1 medium onion, chopped

1 clove garlic or ½ teaspoon garlic salt

6 large white mushrooms, washed and sliced

½ teaspoon thyme

½ teaspoon white pepper

1 teaspoon cornstarch

1½ cups milk or soy milk

2 6-ounce cans of tuna, drained

2 tablespoons grated Parmesan cheese

Cook noodles about 7-10 minutes or until done. Sauté onion, garlic and mushrooms. Add milk and cornstarch with thyme, salt and pepper. Bring to a light boil. Remove and place in a baking dish. Add drained tuna, and mix well. Sprinkle Parmesan cheese and bake in a 350° F. oven for about 25-30 minutes, until heated through.

Vegetable Beef Stir-fry

This is a great way to eat beef since this dish is packed with vegetables. I prefer organic beef since it's lean, tasty and hormone-free. Beef is packed with good protein, B vitamins, B12, zinc and other minerals.

6 8-ounce round steak, lean (cubed)

1 tablespoon olive oil

1 tablespoon soy sauce

1 teaspoon garlic and ginger

1 large onion

1 large red bell pepper

6 ounces snow peas

1 head broccoli, chopped

1 tablespoon cornstarch dissolved in 2 tablespoons cold water

Soy sauce to flavor

Stir-fry beef in olive oil. Add vegetables. Make sauce by combining cornstarch with water; add to mixture and bring to boil. Flavor with soy sauce.

Meat Loaf

Meat loaf is a popular dish, and quite high in protein and easy to make. Serve with my Easy Gravy, page 106 or Barbeque Sauce, page 104 and a green salad with some steamed vegetables.

2-3 pounds ground meat

2 eggs

1 teaspoon salt

¾ cup onion, chopped

½ cup whole wheat-bread crumbs

1 clove garlic

Mix thoroughly and place in oiled loaf pan. Bake one hour at 375° F.

Chapter Twenty-One

Elegant Eggs

According to Dr. Sandra Cabot, in her book, *The Healthy Liver and Bowel Book,* eggs have been mistakenly portrayed as dangerous and unhealthy. But eggs contain high concentrations of valuable nutrients. Most of the studies that show eggs raising cholesterol levels were done with powdered eggs. Powdered eggs contain oxidized or damaged cholesterol known as oxy cholesterol which does raise cholesterol.

Poached, soft or hard-boiled eggs do not raise cholesterol. Cook all eggs with as low heat as possible to prevent further oxidation.

Eggs consumed in moderation are health promoting. Eggs contain lecithin; which helps lower cholesteol and keep it soluble, so it doesn't form plaque in the blood vessels. Eggs contain important amino acids that the liver needs to regulate bile production, and normalize cholesterol levels. If you are concerned, ask your doctor to do a fasting blood test to check the effect of your eating eggs. Dr. Calbot believes that liver function has a greater effect on cholesterol levels than does a modest consumption of healthy foods containing cholesterol.

Basic Omelette

For many people omelettes make a great, nourishing breakfast, especially if cooked with low-heat. I love the free-range and farm-fresh eggs. In regular grocery stores, buy the Eggland's best variety where the chickens have been fed healthy omega 3 fats. Yum!

2 eggs

Dash salt

1 teaspoon butter

Combine salt and eggs and gently beat. Melt butter in pan with low heat. Pour egg mixture into pan. Cook 1 minute or until sides and bottom are set; flip over one side on top of other side. If you want to add vegetables, add them to the egg mixture before you cook the eggs. If you want to add cheese, place it on top of the half-cooked omelette before turning. Serve over sliced whole-grain bread or bagel.

Garden vegetable omelette: Add chopped broccoli, tomato, and onion.

Spinach omelette: Add 1 clove garlic, ¼ cup chopped onions, and ¼ cup chopped spinach.

Cheese omelette: Add ¼ cup grated cheese of choice.

Deviled Eggs

A common picnic food, deviled eggs also make a great meal or quick snack. I like to make it with a healthier, non-hydrogenated type of mayonnaise.

4 hard boiled eggs, cut in half and separate yolks

1 tablespoon mayonnaise (I use Nayonaise)

1 tablespoon Dijon mustard (I like Westbrae)

Dash of each: salt, onion powder and garlic powder

¼ teaspoon paprika for garnish

Remove yolks from egg and put in small bowl and set aside. Mash yolks. Add remaining ingredients (except garnish and egg whites) and stir well to combine. Fill each egg half with yolk mixture. Sprinke with paprika and serve.

Poached Eggs

In a small sauce pan, put a small amount of butter and crack an egg. Add water and simmer 4-5 minutes, or until the yolk changes color from orange to pink and the white is firm. Sprinkle with bread crumbs, grated cheese or salsa to serve.

Eggs Fritata

Another quick way to enjoy eggs.

4 eggs

1 onion, thinly sliced

6 mushrooms, sliced

½ teaspoon salt and a dash of pepper

2 teaspoons butter

3 tablespoons Parmesan cheese

Sauté onion and mushrooms in butter until brown. Set aside. Put eggs, salt and pepper in a bowl and beat. Add onions, mushrooms and mix together. Add remaining butter to the skillet and pour in egg mixture. Fry on top of stove until the mixture settles. Sprinkle Parmesan cheese and broil a few minutes until brown. Cut in wedges and serve.

Eggs Benedict

These are fun for special occasions, but I've made the ingredients healthier. Try this for your next celebration brunch.

Six halves of whole-wheat bagels or bread

Sliced turkey (I prefer organic)

Poached eggs

White sauce (See page 107)

Place the bagel or bread on the plate and cover with a slice of turkey, one egg, and cover with sauce.

Egg Salad

4 hard-boiled eggs, cooled and chopped

¼ cup chopped onion

¼ cup chopped celery

¼ teaspoon each: salt and white pepper

2 tablespoons Dijon mustard

¼ cup mayonnaise (or Tofu mayonnaise or Nayonaise)

Combine all ingredients. Spread on two pieces of whole-grain bread with lettuce.

Scrambled Eggs

Really great. They can be flavored as you like.

4 eggs

2 large garlic cloves, minced

salt to taste

1 small onion, or two thin green onions, minced

1 tablespoon olive oil

Beat eggs; stir in spices and onions. In a skillet, add the olive oil and scramble the egg mixture with a spatula until done. A nice option is to add one tablespoon chopped black olives for taste and color.

Huevos Rancheos

This is a traditional Spanish dish where the eggs are poached and served with a sauce.

Use the above recipe for scrambled eggs; top with salsa or pico de gallo sauce, or grated cheese.

Chapter Twenty-two

Great Grains

Grains don't need to be presoaked, although they should be rinsed before cooking. As with beans, add salt to grain after cooking since they don't cook as well when presalted. Grains are cooked when all of the cooking liquid is absorbed. But taste them. If they are crunchy, they are undercooked. If they are mushy, they are overcooked.

Grains can often be interchangeable. For example, you can substitute brown rice for other varieties of rice and millet.

How do you use grains? The most common form is to boil or bake grains to thoroughly cook the grain. But grains are versatile. Here are some ideas:

As grains:

In soups	In salads
In loaves	In burgers
In cereals	In bean dishes
In vegetable dishes	In breads
As sprouts in salads	Sprouted-wheat bread
As poultry stuffings	

As stuffings for peppers, or cabbage rolls

As flour:

In cereals, pasta, muffins, crackers, English muffins, pancakes, waffles, bagels, noodles, crackers, tortillas, chapati bread, and desserts.

Cooking Grains

Usually you cook one part grain to two parts of water, but some grains vary slightly. Try not to lift the lid while cooking grains, since that will cause the grains to undercook.

One cup	Water	Cooking Time	Yield
Amaranth	11/2 cups	20 minutes	2 cups
Barley	3 cups	11/2 hours	31/2 cups
Basmati	21/2 cups	20 minutes	3 cups
Brown Rice	2 cups	55-60 minutes	3 cups
Buckwheat	2 cups	15 minutes	21/2 cups
Bulgur	2 cups	20 minutes	21/2 cups
Cornmeal	4 cups	25 minutes	3 cups
Couscous	2 cups	15 minutes	23/4 cups
Cracked			
wheat	2 cups	25 minutes	21/3 cups
Kamut	3 cups	40 minutes	2 cups
Millet	2 cups	30-40 minutes	31/2 cups
Oats	2 cups	1 hour	21/2 cups
Quinoa	2 cups	15 minutes	3 cup
Spelt	11/2 cups	30-40 minutes	2 cups
Whole rye	21/2 cups	2 hours	31/4 cups
Whole			
wheat	21/4 cups	13/4 hours	21/2 cups
Wild rice	21/2 cups	1 hour	31/2 cups

Basic Brown Rice

An easy recipe for perfect rice if you don't lift the lid while cooking.

1 cup brown rice

2 cups water

Wash, rinse and drain rice. Put rice in a saucepan and add water. Bring water to a boil, low heat and simmer, covered for 55 minutes.

Variations:

For nutty rice: Add ¼ cup almonds or cashews

For Spanish rice: Add 1 teaspoon Italian seasoning

For Cajun rice: Add 3 tablespoon paprika, 2 teaspoon each white pepper and onion powder, 1 teaspoon oregano and ½ teaspoon cayenne

For breakfast brown rice: Add 1 cup raisins or dates

For curried brown rice: Add ¼ teaspoon curry powder, and ¼ teaspoon turmeric

For cashew rice: Add ¼ cup cashews and raisins

Oatmeal

Oatmeal is a wonderful grain for breakfast, since it's a complex carbohydrate it will stick to your ribs and hold you over until lunch. My friend, Michelle makes a convenient "oatmeal station" in her kitchen. She mixes up the dry ingredients so she can take it with her and eat at her desk before work.

½-¾ cup rolled oats

1½ cups water

½ cup raisins

½ teaspoon cinnamon

Bring water to a boil, add oats and raisins, cinnamon, salt and reduce heat to low, simmering 5-10 minutes or until thick. Serve hot with soy milk, rice milk, honey or maple syrup.

Variations: Substitute ½ cup dates for raisins.

Oriental Wild Rice

This is great! Brown rice and wild rice team up for a wonderfully-flavored rice/vegetable dish. Serve with a salad and whole-grain bread.

Vegetable spray

1 onion, chopped

2 stalks celery, chopped

½ cup mushrooms, sliced

3 cups water or vegetable stock

1 cup cooked brown rice

½ cup wild rice

1 teaspoon salt

Dash of cayenne pepper

1 teaspoon soy sauce

Sauté onion, celery and mushrooms in a saucepan sprayed with vegetable spray a few minutes. Add liquid, rice and salt and bring to a boil. Lower heat and simmer 20 minutes. Add cooked brown rice and heat. Flavor with soy sauce.

Almond Mushroom Rice

Oriental dishes use almonds, mushrooms and rice quite often. Here's a delicious blend that makes a great side dish.

2 cups short-grain brown rice

3 cups water

2 onions, chopped

½ cup slivered almonds

Pinch of thyme

2 cups mushrooms, sliced on diagonal

Wash rice well and drain. Add water and rest of ingredients. Cover and simmer on stove for 50-55 minutes. Stir gently and garnish with parsley sprigs.

Spanish Brown Rice

A traditional dish made healthy. For more convenience, use a salt-free Mexican seasoning in place of the individual herbs and spices.

1¼ cups short-grain brown rice

Pam spray

2 cloves garlic, minced

½ cup onion, chopped

1 green pepper, chopped

2 tomatoes, chopped

2 cups water

1 teaspoon each: paprika, cumin, chili, basil

¼ teaspoon oregano

Dash of cayenne and salt to taste

Wash rice in cold water until water is clear and drain. In the meantime, lightly spray a 2-or 3-quart saucepan with Pam and lightly sauté onion and garlic for 3 minutes. Add brown rice, vegetables, water and spices and allow to come to a boil. Then reduce heat, cover and simmer approximately 50-55 minutes. Don't lift lid while cooking since this will increase cooking time and rice will become soggy.

Wild Rice Stuffing

This can be used as a stuffing or as a great side dish.

Vegetable spray

1 onion, chopped

2 stalks celery, chopped

½ cup mushrooms, sliced

3 cups water or vegetable stock

2 cups cooked brown rice (1 cup brown rice cooked 50 minutes in 2 cups water)

1 cup wild rice (1 cup dry cooked 30 minutes in 1¼ cups water)

1 teaspoon salt

Dash of cayenne pepper

1 teaspoon soy sauce

1 tablespoon rosemary

1 teaspoon thyme

1 tablespoon sage

Optional: nuts

Sauté onion, celery and mushrooms in a saucepan sprayed with vegetable spray a few minutes.   Add liquid, wild rice and salt and bring to a boil. Lower heat and simmer 20 minutes. Add cooked brown rice and spices and warm.

Stuffed Cabbage Rolls

Want to fix cabbage in ways that kids like? Here's an easy dish that's fun to eat. But don't stop here. Cabbage lends itself to many types of stuffings: bean, grain or vegetables.

1 cabbage (6-8 leaves)

Filling:

Vegetable spray

¼ cup minced onion

1 10-ounce package frozen chopped spinach

2 cups mixed cooked brown and wild rice (Lundberg Wild Blend)

Salt to taste (½ teaspoon)

½ teaspoon Frontier Five-Spice Powder (or cinnamon, fennel, cloves, anise, pepper)

5-6 tablespoons dried potato flakes

Optional: 1 teaspoon olive oil

Remove center core from a head of cabbage. Gently remove the leaves one at a time. If the leaves are hard to take off, then poor hot water over them or steam the entire head and remove leaves. Cut away the core from each leaf. Steam the cabbage leaves until they are soft, about 5-8 minutes.

Filling: Sauté the onion in a saucepan coated with vegetable spray. Add the spinach, brown rice and wild rice, salt and add five-spice powder and mix well. Add the potato flakes and olive oil if desired. To stuff, place leaves flat and put 1/3 cup of stuffing on each cabbage leaf. Fold both sides toward the middle and roll up, starting at core end of each leaf, and roll away from you. Secure with a toothpick.

You can pour a cooked tomato sauce over these, or place

each of the cabbage rolls in a casserole dish, pour a tomato sauce over, and bake for 5 minutes in a 350° F. oven.

Variations: Try other cooked grains like quinoa, millet, or kasha, or even tempeh for filling.

Old Fashioned Museli

A traditional Swiss breakfast, it's often made with yogurt which makes it a bit runny. Here's a delicious version.

3 tablespoons quick-cooking oats

1½ tablespoons wheat germ

2 tablespoons sunflower seeds or cashews, chopped

2 tablespoons chopped almonds

2 tablespoons raisins

1 tablespoon oat bran

2 tablespoons date or maple sugar

Mix above ingredients together and store in a container. Use as a cold cereal, or heat with 1 cup water for a hot cereal. Simmer on low 2-3 minutes. Enjoy with milk, soy or rice milk.

Chapter Twenty-three

Pasta Dishes

P asta is a staple food around the world which has been used for centuries. Made from flour, water and sometimes eggs, pasta can come in many varieties and styles: lasagne, elbowl, angel hair, spaghetti, linguine, fetucine, shells, ziti, rigatoni, rotini, spirals, ribbon, orzo, egg noodles, vermicelli, cannelloni, and manicoti.

Pasta can be made from: whole wheat, quionoa, spelt, brown rice, kamut, artichoke, buckwheat, corn, and oat flours. However, many pastas are made from the refined part of the wheat kernel which is called the endosperm, or starch which contains no fiber and few minerals. Buckwheat pasta, also called soba is made from buckwheat flour and sometimes contains wheat. Mung bean starch pastas are highly refined which makes them so quick cooking. Ramen style noodles like those made by Westbrae are nutritious, often made from brown rice, buckwheat or wheat. Pasta should only be eaten once a week, with portion control.

Pasta and Cheese

This is a quick healthy version of Macaroni and Cheese and a great dish for dinner or company.

One package whole-wheat pasta

1 cup firm tofu

½ cup grated Parmesan cheese

¼ teaspoon garlic powder

¼ teaspoon paprika

2 tablespoons dried chives

¼ cup butter (or Spectrum Spread)

Optional: ¼ cup Romano cheese

Cook ribbons according to package. Blend tofu in blender or food processor until smooth. Combine tofu and seasonings while ribbon pasta cooks. Drain ribbon pasta. Stir in ¼ cup butter or Spectrum Spread. Add cheese mixture to ribbons and cook over low heat until cheese is melted and mixture becomes thick, approximately 5 to 7 minutes.

Linguine in Mushroom Sauce

This sauce is great over pasta, especially linguine.

1 cup mushrooms, sliced

1 clove garlic, minced

1 14-ounce can artichoke hearts

3 teaspoons ripe olives, sliced

Salt

1 tablespoon cornstarch or arrowroot powder

1 cup water

1 package linguine

Mix together mushrooms, artichoke hearts, olives and salt. Mix cornstarch in water and add to mixture. Heat until thick. Serve over cooked linguine.

To cook linguine, follow directions on package.

Tofu Lasagna

This is a great substitute for high-fat lasagnes, and was a great hit with the classes. Be sure to find a tomato sauce that you enjoy. You can add spinach or other vegetables, too.

Pam olive oil cooking spray

1 onion, minced

4 cloves garlic, minced

1 bunch leeks, chopped

8 white mushrooms, sliced

¼ teaspoon dried parsley

1 teaspoon salt

¼ cup Parmesan Cheese

1 19-ounce block Silken Tofu, mashed

1 8-ounce package Mozzarella

1 26-ounce jar pasta sauce

Lasagna noodles

Preheat oven to 375° F. **For filling:** Lightly spray a saucepan with vegetable spray and sauté onion and garlic until translucent. Add sliced leeks, parsley and mushrooms and cook a few minutes. Add salt and Parmesan cheese, and tofu. Mix well and set aside. Shred the cheese and put aside. Meanwhile, cook lasagna noodles, drain and rinse in cold water. Then lightly spray a 9 x 13" baking dish.

To assemble: Lay three lasagna noodles in pan. Then spread half of the tofu mixture over the noodles. Then layer half of the Tofu Rella on top of the tofu mixture. Then spoon half of the tomato sauce over the tofu mixture. Repeat layers once again ending with sauce. Bake uncovered at 375° F for 30 minutes. Traditionally, lasagna is high in fat because of the meat and cheeses. This recipe is dairy free except for the Parmesan cheese and is considerably lower in fat. You can make this with your favorite pasta sauce with meat and it will still be lower in fat because of using tofu instead of high-fat cheeses.

Variations: Add ½ cup spinach or broccoli/carrot and lentil mixture.

Note: If you are allergic to tomatoes, then try a sauce using carrots instead of tomatoes. Cut up carrots, and sauté with onion and garlic and use the same spices as in the tomato sauce.

Fettucini With Marinara Sauce

Another hit with the classes. The Marina sauce has no fat.

Olive oil
1 onion, chopped
2 carrots, chopped
4 cups tomatoes, chopped (2 pounds or 4-5 tomatoes)
1 teaspoon each: basil and oregano
½ teaspoon garlic powder
Salt to taste
1 package fettucini

Marinara Sauce: Sauté onion until translucent in a saucepan lightly sprayed with vegetable spray. Add carrots, tomatoes and spices. Cover and cook 20 minutes. Take out half of mixture and puree in blender or food processor. Return to pot, heat and serve hot. (If you desire to thicken sauce, add 2-3 tablespoon tomato paste or 1 tablespoon corn meal.)

Fettucini: In a large pot of water, cook fettucini 4-5 minutes until done. Add one tablespoon of oil to keep pasta from sticking.) Do not overcook. Drain, but don't rinse.

Pour Marinara Sauce over Pasta. Serve with side green salad and garlic bread.

Chinese Noodles With Thai Angel Hair Pasta

If you can get a spicy pasta, even better.

1 tablespoon soy sauce

2 tablespoons olive oil

2 tablespoons brown rice vinegar

2 teaspoons ginger root powder

1 cup of peas or snow peas (fresh or frozen)

1 yellow or red pepper, sliced in thin strips

One package angel hair pasta

Chinese Sauce: In a bowl, combine soy sauce, oil, vinegar and ginger root powder. Use raw (or quickly steam or sauté snow peas and pepper slices in small sauce pan.) Add to oil/vinegar mixture.

Pasta: Cook pasta 2-3 minutes in a large pot of boiling water. (One tablespoon of oil added will keep pasta from sticking.) Do not overcook. Drain, but don't rinse. Pour Chinese Sauce with vegetables over pasta and toss. Serve with baked chicken and broccoli/carrot side dish.

Low-Fat Pesto With Linguine

I've tried to make a pesto that was low-fat, and here's what I came up with:

¼ cup dried basil (or ¾ cup fresh)

1 cup fresh parsley

3 tablespoons Parmesan cheese

3 cloves garlic, minced

4-6 tablespoons slivered almonds

1 tablespoon white miso paste

¾-1 cup water

2 tablespoons olive oil

One package linguine

Pesto: Combine all ingredients except water and oil in a blender or food processor and process until smooth. Add water, a little at a time until desired consistency. Add the oil last.

Linguine: Cook linguine 5-7 minutes in a large pot of boiling water. (One tablespoon of oil added will keep pasta from sticking.) Do not overcook. Drain, but don't rinse. Spoon Pesto over linguine. Serve with baked Italian chicken, garlic bread and side dish of sautéed onions and zucchini.

Wild Rice and Bowtie Pasta

3 tablespoons olive oil

½ cup broccoli (frozen or fresh)

½ cup green, red or yellow pepper slices

½ cup carrot slices

1 cup cooked bowtie pasta

1 cup cooked wild rice

Seasoning: In a separate bowl, add 3 tablespoon olive oil, stir well and let stand. Use raw, steamed or sautéed broccoli, carrots and peppers. Add to seasoning mixture and set aside. Meanwhile, cook Bowtie pasta and wild rice in a large pot of water over medium heat. (One tablespoon of oil added will keep pasta from sticking.) Do not overcook. Don't rinse. Drain and toss pasta with seasoning mixture. Season to taste. Serve with side green salad and whole-wheat rolls.

Variation: Add 1 cup chopped turkey or crumbled Tofu Ground Round.

Italian Pasta

This can make a nice meal if you add some chicken or other protein.

2 cups cooked pasta of choice

1 cup frozen green beans/corn mix

1 can red beans, drained

¼ cup vinegar

1 clove garlic, or dash garlic salt

1 teaspoon Italian seasonings

½ cup silken firm tofu

Optional: 1 teaspoon honey

Lemon juice to taste

Optional: 1-2 tablespoons sliced almonds or slivers

Optional: 6-7 grilled chicken strips

Cook pasta according to directions, drain and cool. Combine cooked pasta, vegetables and beans in a large salad bowl. Make dressing in a separate bowl or blender with vinegar, garlic, Italian seasoning, tofu and honey. Mix well and pour over salad and serve, garnishing with a few sliced almonds.

Oriental Pasta

This was a hit, in the cooking classes, too.

2 cups cooked garlic angel hair pasta

2 thin carrots, cut in rounds

1 cup green beans or snap peas

1 yellow squash, cut on rounds

½ can water chestnuts, drained

1 cucumber

Dressing:

¼ cup raspberry wine vinegar or apple cider vinegar

1 tablespoon sesame seed

1 tablespoon soy sauce

1 teaspoon brown sugar or Sucanat

Dash of cayenne pepper

1 tablespoon sesame seeds for garnish

Combine ingredients in a large salad bowl: cooked pasta, carrots, green beans or snap peas, yellow squash, water chestnuts and cucumber.

Make dressing in a separate bowl or blender. Mix well and pour over salad and serve, garnishing with sesame seeds.

Chapter Twenty-four

Breads, Muffins and Pancakes

Virtually every grain and many types of beans can be ground on stone mills into flour. Wheat flour is perhaps the most popular flour for baking, since wheat is high in gluten which makes bread sticky and hold together. To make the best tasting bread, you need to use the highest quality ingredients.

Bread is simply made from flour, salt and water. Adding yeast causes the bread to rise which makes a lighter bread. There are two steps: first dissolve the yeast, and then add flour, salt and water to the yeast mixture. Knead, let rise and bake and enjoy. But eat bread and bread products moderately.

Basic Whole-Wheat Bread

There's nothing like a loaf of freshly-baked homemade bread! This is a basic loaf that can be used to make dinner rolls, pizza crust, cinnamon rolls, or foccacia bread.

A drop of honey

2 tablespoons yeast dissolved in ½ cup warm water

(110° F.)

2 cups lukewarm water

¼ cup honey

¼ cup olive oil

1 teaspoon salt

3 tablespoons wheat gluten or ¼ cup gluten flour

3 cups whole-wheat flour

3 cups unbleached white flour*

***I prefer a darker, heavier bread so I usually use 6 cups of whole-wheat flour**

1. Dissolve yeast in water and add just a drop or so of honey for about 5 minutes, which is called proofing the yeast. If the yeast is too old, it won't bubble. If it's fresh, it will foam up and bubble. The water should be about 100-110 ° F. If it's too hot, over 120° F, it will kill the yeast, but if it's too cold, the yeast won't work. It has to be just right! A kitchen thermometer will help. Adding a drop of honey feeds the yeast. You can use malt, maple syrup, molasses, or rice syrup.

*For best results, have all ingredients at room temperature, and be sure the yeast water is warm enough.

In a large bowl, mix together the water, oil, honey, salt and yeast mixture. Add the gluten flour or Vital Wheat Gluten and 3 cups of whole-wheat flour. Beat with a wooden spoon about 100 strokes, which activates the gluten which makes a lighter bread. Add more flour as necessary to make a kneadable dough.

Oil makes the bread tender, but you can either decrease the oil, or omit it.

Honey will feed the yeast and also flavor the bread, although you can decrease the amount if desired.

Salt helps to flavor the bread and helps to digest bread.

Wheat gluten helps to make a light-textured, spongier bread. However, it's an optional ingredient.

Whole-wheat flour has the greatest amount of gluten and yields the best bread. Dough should not be sticky.

2. Turn dough on a well-floured surface and knead enough to make a smooth dough that is not sticky.

The best is to knead about 400-600 times. Generally, the more you knead, the better. Continue kneading until the dough feels smooth and satiny, which can take about 20 minutes.

3. Place the kneaded dough in a large, oiled bowl (to keep the dough from sticking to it). Oil the top of the dough. Cover the bowl with a clean, damp cloth and let sit in a warm place until the dough doubles. Punch down. The ideal temperature is about 80-85° F.; the lower the temp, the longer it will take to rise. You can let it rise a second time, but this is not necessary. It makes a lighter loaf, though.

4. Cut the dough in half. Shape one half of the dough into a loaf and put in well oiled loaf pan, 4 ½ x 8 ½. Bake at 350° F. for 45 minutes. Don't preheat the oven since the bread will rise more before beginning to bake. Let cool 10-15 minutes before slicing. Let cool completely before wrapping.

5. For the other half of the dough, follow directions below for Foccacia bread. It makes about a dozen dinner rolls, or 2 bread loaves, or one bread and one foccacia loaf.

Focaccia Bread

Topping:

1 large onion

5 cloves of garlic

¼ teaspoon salt

½ to 1 teaspoon Herbes de Provence

1. Oil a round pizza pan. Press the dough out until it covers the sheet or pan.

2. Make the topping. Sauté the onion and garlic and spices. Cool. Then poke small holes in the dough. Lightly spread some oil on the dough and then spread the topping on the dough.

3. Bake at 350° F. for about 20 minutes. Serve hot, cut in squares.

Other breads that you can make from this basic dough: dinner rolls, pizza dough, or cinnamon rolls.

Dinner rolls: After your bread has risen, then punch it down and pull off small pieces of bread, about 1-2 inches thick. Roll into rounds, and if you like, roll these balls into seeds (poppy, sesame or sunflower). You may need to squirt with water for the seeds to stick to the dough. Place on an oiled baking sheet and bake at 350° F. for about 20 minutes.

Pizza dough: Press the dough out until it covers the sheet or pan. Now place small prick holes in the bread with a knife or fork. This will keep the bread from rising. Then place toppings on the bread: tomato sauce, onions, peppers, mushrooms, tomatoes, and anything else you like. Top with cheese (I like using soy cheese) and bake for about 30-40 minutes at 350° F.

Cinnamon rolls: Press the dough out until it's flat. Then make a mixture of Sucanat and cinnamon powder and pour over the dough. Then carefully roll the dough up from one side to the other. It will look like a long log. Then cut the log in 3-4 inch segments and separate. You can let these pieces of dough rise for 20 minutes. Then put them on a lightly-oiled sheet and bake at 350° F. for about 30 minutes.

Banana Bread

½ cup brown sugar or Sucanat

¼ cup oil

2 eggs (or egg whites or substitutes)

¼ cup honey

2-3 bananas, mashed

5-6 tablespoons yogurt (or other liquid)

2 cups whole-wheat pastry flour

¾ teaspoon salt

1½ teaspoons baking powder

½ teaspoon soda

Optional: ¼ cup nuts, ground

Combine sugar, oil, eggs, honey, bananas and liquid. In another bowel, combine flour, salt, soda and baking powder. Add the liquid ingredients to dry ingredients. Pour into oiled loaf pan. Bake at 350° F. for 45-50 minutes.

Dill Bread

Here's an easy quick bread. Great with a meal or as a snack.

1 cup corn meal

1 cup whole-wheat flour

1 teaspoon Rumford's baking powder

Dash of salt

3 tablespoon dillweed

¼ cup oil

4 tablespoons honey or maple syrup

1 egg or egg replacer

1 cup milk

Separately, mixed the corn meal, whole-wheat flour, baking powder sea salt and dillweed. In another bowl, mix the wet ingredients: oil, honey, soy milk, and egg. Pour the wet ingredients into the dry ingredients and stir until moist. (If needed, add a small amount of liquid to make a cake-like batter). Pour in a 9" square pan which has been lightly oiled with vegetable spray. Bake at 350° F for approximately 40 minutes. (Lower degree 25 points if using glass bakeware.)

Quick Rye Bread

Rye bread is a traditional food which can be made yeasted, unyeasted or with a sour dough starter. Here's a quick bread.

1½ cups rye flour

1 cup whole-wheat pastry flour

1 teaspoon salt

2½ teaspoons baking powder

1 egg, beaten

1½ cups soy or rice milk

3 tablespoons canola oil

1 onion, chopped and sautéed

1 teaspoon caraway, ground

Preheat oven to 350° F. Mix dry ingredients together. Sauté onion and set aside. In a different bowl, combine the wet ingredients. Add sautéed onions to wet ingredients. Mix wet and dry ingredients and add more liquid if needed. Dough should be somewhat sticky. Form into pan and sprinkle caraway seeds. Bake in a 9 x 5 x 3-inch oiled pan at 350° F. for 55 minutes or until knife comes out clean.

Essene or Manna Bread

This is one of the healthiest breads you can eat, since it's simply wheat berries which have been sprouted. No yeast or sweetener is required. You can find this type of bread from Manna Foods or Lifestream in special food stores or health food stores.

5 cups of wheat berries

Water to cover

Chopped dates or raisins

Soak wheat berries in water for 15-18 hours. Drain. Put in a jar and let sprout for 3 days. Water sprouts twice a day; keep them wet, but not soaked. After sprouting, put sprouts through a grain mill, vitamix or champion juicer. Add dates and raisins. Form into a ball and knead. Spread on an oiled cookie sheet and bake at low heat 240 ° F. for 4 hours or 350° F. for 2 hours.

Variations: Add ½ teaspoon each: garlic, basil, sage, and oregano.

Add ½ teaspoon each: caraway seeds, and dill.

Muffins

A muffin is made from flour, a liquid, a sweetener, and oil. For example, 2 cups of whole-wheat flour plus ¼ cup oil, plus 1 cup soy milk and an egg. Add baking powder, soda and salt will raise and flavor it. For convenience, Arrowhead Mills has a basic bran muffin mix that you add an egg and water to, and any other kind of fruit: apples, a banana, raisins, berries, oranges, carob and so on.

Banana Bran Muffins

These were a hit in the classes and make a nice snack for after school.

1 cup whole-wheat pastry flour

2½ teaspoons Rumford Baking Powder

Pinch salt

1 cup oat bran

½ cup honey

2 tablespoons canola oil or ¼ cup fruit puree

2 eggs or (or egg replacement)

1 cup mashed banana

½ cup apple juice or milk or soy milk

¼ teaspoon vanilla extract

Optional: 1 cup raisins or 1 tablespoon cinnamon

Preheat oven to 400° F. Combine flour, salt, bran and baking powder in a bowl. In another bowl, combine honey, oil, milk, egg or egg replacer. Add the banana and mix well. Combine the wet ingredients with the dry ingredients until well mixed, but don't overmix. Fill oiled muffin tins and bake for 20-25 minutes. Insert a toothpick or knife to check. If done, knife or toothpick will come out clean.

To make bread, decrease temperature to 350° F.; bake at 55-60 minutes in an oiled loaf pan.

Multi-Grain Belgium Waffles

Waffles are a treat on Sunday morning. This recipe is great; the students liked it better than a mix.

2 cups whole wheat flour (or 1 cup whole-wheat flour/1 cup oat or millet flour)

2 teaspoons baking powder

¼ teaspoon salt

1 teaspoon Sucanat

1 to 2 cups milk

1 teaspoon oil

Optional: 1 egg or egg replacer, or ¼ cup pureed fruit

Combine dry ingredients in a bowl. In another bowl, combine liquid ingredients. Blend together. Lightly oil skillet, and pour ¼ batter, cover and cook over low flame 5 minutes. Top with strawberries and tofu whipped cream. (Or, maple syrup, maple/fruit syrup, applesauce, and so on.)

Variations: For extra flavor or variety, try adding cinnamon, raisins, sesame seeds, almond slices, or fruit puree (applesauce, banana puree, pear puree, and so on.)

Tofu Whipped Cream

Okay, so it's not exactly like whipped cream that you know and love! But it's really healthy and actually tastes good!

2 cups tofu

¼ cup honey

1 tablespoon canola oil

¼ teaspoon vanilla

2 tablespoons fructose

Dash sea salt

Blend well in a blender. Use as a topping for waffles or pies or anywhere you would use whipped cream.

Basic Pancakes

1 cup whole-wheat pastry flour

½ cup unbleached white pastry flour

1 cup soy milk or rice milk

1-2 tablespoons olive or canola oil

1 egg or 1 teaspoon egg replacer or two egg whites, or
1 cup blended tofu

1½ teaspoons baking powder

Dash salt

Combine dry ingredients and add wet ingredients. Oil a pan and heat it to medium heat. Use about ¼ cup batter for each pancake. Cook about 1-2 minutes per side. Serve with healthy toppings listed under Belgium Waffles.

French Toast

A simple, healthy recipe.

6 pieces of whole-wheat bread

2 cups of milk

2 eggs

1 tablespoon cinnamon

1-2 tablespoons olive oil

Whisk the milk, flaxseed, eggs, oil and cinnamon. Soak bread until soft. Over medium heat, grill bread on both sides for about 3 minutes, until browned. Top with favorite toppings. Serve immediately.

Chapter Twenty-five

Desserts and Cookies

Desserts are nice on special occasions, but obviously if eaten too frequently, even natural desserts will cause weight gain. One way to eat occasional desserts without too much guilt is to use the best ingredients such as natural sweeteners instead of sugar, or whole-grain flours instead of white flour. Here are some of my favorite desserts.

Banana Yogurt Dessert

1 banana

½ apple

2 tablespoons honey

1 teaspoon vanilla

1 cup tofu or yogurt

Blend. Freeze for 3 hours. Remove, re-blend and serve.

Fruit Sorbet

Yum, tasty, easy, and even elegant enough for a dinner party.

2 cups frozen berries

1 tablespoon honey or maple syrup

2 bananas, sliced

½ teaspoon lemon juice

Blend ingredients and freeze. After 2 hours or so, break up slightly and re-freeze. Serve in a parfait glass.

Healthy Popsicle

What a healthy treat for children. My friend Julianna calls them "great hunger busters."

1 cup black cherries

½ cup frozen concentrate

¼-½ cup water

Process all ingredients in blender or food processor. Pour into molds and freeze. Insert popsicle sticks into mixture when partially frozen.

Brown Rice Pudding

I love rice pudding and was delighted to create a healthier version of this traditional dish.

1½ cups cooked short-grain brown rice

5-6 tablespoons honey

¼ cup raisins

1 cup milk (I like Westsoy non-fat vanilla)

2 teaspoons vanilla extract

1 egg, beaten

1 tablespoon cornstarch or arrowroot, in 1-2 tablespoons water

In a saucepan, combine the rice, honey, raisins, milk, vanilla. Add egg and cornstarch or arrowroot. Bring to a boil, and turn on simmer cooking 10-15 minutes or until thick. If you use regular cow's milk, you may have to sweeten to taste. Vanilla soy milk is already sweet. Let cool and chill. Serve cold, garnish with a slice of strawberry.

Variation: Add 1-2 mashed bananas, or 4 tablespoons baking powder to make lighter.

Easy and Quick Tofu Chocolate Pudding

You can't make a dessert quicker or easier than this healthy pudding.

10 ounces tofu, firm

½ cup Wonderslim 99.9% caffeine free cocoa

¼ cup fructose

2 tablespoons cup water

Blend together and spoon into custard cups or bowl. Chill. Top with slivered almonds, strawberries, or sliced bananas.

I have experimented with other sweeteners. If you use honey, omit the water. Date sugar is delicious, but it gives the pudding a slightly gritty taste. Stevia doesn't work. Sucanat would be nice, but is not as sweet. Fructose works best.

Apple Pie

A healthier version of an American classic.

Crust:

1 cup whole wheat-pastry flour and 1 cup unbleached white-pastry flour*

½-¾ cup canola oil or Spectrum Spread (non-hydrogenated)

Dash of salt

7-9 tablespoons cold water

This recipe makes 2 crusts, one for top and one for bottom. To make a single crust, cut the recipe in half. Mix flour and oil until well combined and crumbly, using a wire whisk. Add sea salt. Slowly add cold water, a tablespoon at a time until dough forms a ball. Roll out on a floured surface. Place in a standard pie plate.

Filling:

6 apples, peeled and chopped

1 teaspoon cinnamon

¼ teaspoon nutmeg

2 tablespoons whole-wheat pastry flour

¾ cup brown sugar or Sucanat

Dash salt

Combine apples, spices, flour and sugar in a large bowl. Place in pie. Roll out top layer of crust and place on top of pie, making design slits (or, roll out and cut strips to make a lattice over pie.) Bake at 375° F. for 50-55 minutes. Let cool and serve.

Variations: Other flour combinations are: ½ part oat flour ½ part whole-wheat pastry flour; or ½ part oat flour and ½ part unbleached-white pastry flour, or ½ part quick cooking oats and ½ part whole-wheat pastry flour. Another combination is just using brown rice flour or oat flour alone.

Variation: Use 1 cup whole-wheat pastry flour, and ½ cup brown rice flour or ½ cup whole-wheat pastry flour and ½ cup millet. Both make a nice pie crust, but are not strong enough to stand alone.

Variation: To sweeten pie without brown sugar use ¼ teaspoon stevia powder or ½ cup brown rice syrup.

For lower fat content, substitute one part of oil for one part unsweetened applesauce.

Easy Cherry Pie

I loved to bake pies growing up, especially apple and cherry pies. This pie is delightful and so easy to make.

Pie crust (see page 219)

1 12-ounce bag frozen dark cherries

1 teaspoon cornstarch

1 cup water

½ cup brown sugar

In a saucepan, combine cherries, cornstarch, water and brown sugar and bring to a slight boil. Place in pie crust. Bake at 350° F. for about 30-40 minutes. Serve with non-fat vanilla frozen yogurt.

Pumpkin Pie

Crust: 1 box Health Valley Date Cookies, fruit
sweetened

Filling: 2 cups cooked mashed pumpkin puree (or 1
can pumpkin pie filling)

½ cup milk

2 eggs, or egg whites (fresh or powder), beaten
(or ½ pound blended tofu or yogurt)

½ cup honey

1 teaspoon cinnamon

½ teaspoon ginger

¼ teaspoon nutmeg

¼ teaspoon ground cloves

Filling: Combine the pumpkin, sweetener, milk, eggs and spices in a bowl. Mix well and pour into pie shell. Using tofu or yogurt in place of eggs makes a softer pie, not as firm as with eggs.

Pie Shell:

1½ cup whole-wheat pastry flour

3 tablespoons oil or Spectrum Spread

Dash salt

5-6 tablespoons cold water

Mix flour and oil until well combined and crumbly. Add salt. Slowly add water, a tablespoon at a time until the dough forms a ball. Don't overwork. Roll out on a floured surface. Put in pie pan and flute edges. Bake at 350° F. for 10 minutes. Pour pumpkin mix into pie shells. Bake at 375° F. for 1 hour or until knife comes out clean when inserted. Let cool and serve.

Quick Easy, Pie Shell: An easy way to make a pie shell is to use a box of Health Valley fat-free cookies. Crush cookies or crumble in a coffee mill. Wet hands and press cookie crumbles in a 9" pie dish, no more than halfway up the sides. Fill pie and bake at 350 F. for one hour.

Chocolate Chip Nut Cookies

Both Carol's and Vicki's families enjoyed these delicious treats. You can substitute carob chips for chocolate chips.

½-¾ cup honey

½ cup butter or spectrum spread (or 1 cup applesauce or equivalent of mashed banana)

½ cup Sucanat (or other sugar: date sugar, maple sugar, fructose

¼ cup milk powder or milk substitute

1 egg, beaten or egg replacer

2 tablespoons cornstarch

1 teaspoon vanilla

1 cup whole-wheat flour

½ cup oat bran

¾ cup chocolate or carob chips (non-dairy is best)

½ whole-wheat pastry flour or unbleached white
flour

½ cup chopped almonds (or pecans)

Mix dry ingredients and add to mixed liquid ingredients.
Fold in carob chips and almonds. Drop a spoonful or two of
batter on a cookie sheet sprayed with vegetable spray. Bake
10-12 minutes at 350° F. oven or until very lightly browned.
Makes 2-3 dozen cookies. To make bar cookies, spread the
batter ½ inch thick on a cookie sheet and bake at 350° F. for
15-20 minutes. Cook and cut into squares or bars.

Oatmeal Raisin Cookies

¼ cup canola oil

1¾ cup soy milk or low-fat milk

1 egg or egg substitute

½ teaspoon vanilla

1½ cups whole-wheat flour (50/50)

1½ cups rolled oats

½ cup brown sugar or Sucanat

¼ teaspoon salt

1 teaspoon baking powder

1 cup raisins

Preheat oven to 350° F. Mix dry ingredients (sugar, flour,
oats, salt, baking powder) separately from wet ingredients
(oil, milk, egg and vanilla.) Mix wet ingredients with dry and

add raisins. Drop by tablespoonful on an oiled cookie sheet and flatten. Bake for 10 minutes until slightly brown. Makes 2-3 dozen depending on the size.

Peanut Butter Cookies

Trying to make a "low-fat" peanut butter cookie is a contradiction, isn't it? But I have found a way to make these lower in fat, by cutting the peanut butter to ½ cup, omitting extra oil, and making a flavorful, cake-like cookie that people really like.

2¼ cups flour (part whole wheat pastry and part unbleached white flour)

½ teaspoon each baking soda and baking powder

¼ teaspoon salt

1 cup granulated sugar (fructose, sucanat, etc.)

½ cup unhydrogenated peanut butter

2 eggs or egg replacer or egg whites

1 cup soy or other milk

Mix dry ingredients in one bowl and then wet ingredients in a separate bowl, beating the eggs or egg whites well. Combine all ingredients together and mix well. Form into small 1" balls. Place on ungreased cookie sheet and flatten with a fork crosswise. Bake at 350° F. for 10 minutes. Cool. Makes 3 dozen.

Chapter Twenty-Six

Party Beverages and Desserts

The beverages and desserts in this section are the types of recipes that you would want to make for special occasions since they are a bit richer in flavor and take longer to make. I included several cheesecake recipes too.

Herbal Tea Holiday Punch

Many herbal teas make a wonderful base for a nice punch and most blend well with fruits and fruit juices. Celestial Seasonings and Republic of Tea have a variety of teas that can make an infinite number of punches.

1 can frozen apple juice concentrate

1 liter sparkling water

6-7 bags of brewed Herbal Tea

crushed ice

Steep tea and remove bags. Add fruit juice concentrate and sparkling water. Mix well and serve cold with crushed ice.

Healthy Party Punch

I've looked for alternatives to the sugar-sweetened punches and came up with a wonderful punch that keeps people coming back for more.

Variation: *For added enjoyment, in the punch, float 1-2 cups of frozen fruit or a healthy fruit sorbet (found at your health food store).*

2 cups white grape juice

2 cups apple juice

2 cups sparkling water

Optional: 1 cup frozen strawberries or a 1-3 cups fruit sorbet

Mix together and chill. Adding frozen fruit or a sorbet keeps this punch cold. Garnish with strawberry or lemon wedge. This is a nice for parties.

My Delicious Hot Chocolate Drink

You can make a chocolate drink with cocoa powder, milk and a sweetener. I like using Wonderslim's 99% caffeine-free cocoa powder, but you could substitute carob powder. This recipe is great when you want a hot drink similar to hot chocolate without the caffeine and extra fat. I experimented with various milk alternatives and they all taste great in this drink. The coffee substitute adds more flavor.

1 cup milk of choice

1 tablespoon honey or sweetener of choice

1 tablespoon caffeine-free cocoa or carob powder

1 tablespoon Kafix or coffee substitute

Mix together in a sauce pan, over low heat and stir gently. Serve hot.

Healthy Eggnog

Like many of my clients, I grew up drinking eggnog at Christmas. But we wanted to enjoy the taste of eggnog without the fat and sugar. I experimented with an eggless eggnog for my clients who are allergic to eggs. Here it is!

2 cups soy milk

2 bananas

1 teaspoon vanilla

¼ teaspoon nutmeg

Optional: ¼ cup tofu

Mix ingredients and blend well. Serve cold. Garnish with a sprinkle of nutmeg on top.

Hot Holiday Cider

Here's a nice cider that has less sugar than usual and tastes great.

1 quart apple cider or apple juice

2-3 cloves

1 stick cinnamon

2 tablespoons lemon juice

2 tablespoons orange juice

This recipe can be served hot or cold. Heat cider or juice and add spices. When warm, add lemon and orange juice. Remove cloves and cinnamon stick. Serve warm, or add ice and serve chilled. For added carbonation, add spritzer or sparkling water.

Strawberry Cheesecake

Cheesecake is traditionally high in fats, up to 33 grams of fat for one slice. This cheesecake is fat free! You can substitute 2 cups of yogurt cheese for the sour cream and cream cheese. To make yogurt cheese, drain the liquid off of plain yogurt, using a strainer with a cheese cloth or coffee filter. Drain in refrigerator for 12 hours for whipped cream cheese consistency or 24 hours for cream cheese consistency which is best for cheese cake recipes.

This cheesecake is one of the richest that I've made. It has a wonderful flavor, texture and color using the Soya Kasa soy cream cheese or the fat-reduced cream cheese. Both are preferable to the fat-free varieties. While this cheesecake is slightly higher in fat grams, it's also one of the best "healthy" cheesecakes I've made. Great for a special occasion.

One box Health Valley Fat-free cookies (Hawaiian, Apricot or Date)

2 containers fat-reduced cream cheese or Soya Kaas tofu cream cheese

2 eggs, or 2 egg whites, or equivalent egg substitute

½-¾ cup sugar, fructose or date sugar

2 tablespoons oat flour or pastry flour

1 teaspoon lemon juice

1 teaspoon vanilla extract

15-20 strawberries, sliced

Coat a 9-inch springform pan with nonstick vegetable spray. Crumble Health Valley Fat-free cookies in the bottom of the pan. Bake at 350° F. for 6-7 minutes or until the edges are firm and lightly brown. Set aside.

Place the cream cheese, and eggs or egg substitute in a food processor or blender and blend until smooth. Mix the sugar and flour together and add to cream cheese mixture. Add the vanilla and lemon juice and blend until smooth. Spread into pie crust. Bake at 325° F. for 45-55 minutes. (Bake in middle of the oven.) Let cool 30 minutes and chill. After chilled, place sliced strawberries around the edges of the cheesecake. Put about a cup of strawberries in a blender with 1-2 teaspoons of fructose or a dash of stevia and blend. Drizzle across each piece as you serve the cheesecake. For best results, chill a few hours before serving.

For amaretto cheesecake: Add 1 teaspoon almond extract to basic recipe and omit the strawberries.

Tofu Cheesecake

This is a great way to enjoy tofu and a delicious dessert.

Crust:

2 cups rolled oats

2 cups wheat germ

½ cups olive oil

¼ cup honey

½ teaspoon salt

Combine all ingredients and pat into a 9 x 13 size baking pan and bake at 350° F. until brown (just a few minutes).

Filling:

1 16-ounce carton firm tofu

½ cup honey

3 tablespoons lemon juice

2 tablespoons vanilla

¼ cup whole-wheat pastry flour

3 tablespoons cornstarch

2 tablespoons fructose

1 banana

Filling: Combine all ingredients and blend in blender until creamy. Pour filling over prepared crust. Bake in over at 350° F. for 5 minutes. Cool. Top with Tofu Whipped Cream, page 212 or Stevia Whipped Cream (below) and sliced bananas or strawberries.

Stevia Whipped Cream

A great topping.

Dash of stevia powder

1 pint whipped cream

Blend well and serve.

Better Butter

1 teaspoon stevia powder

½ cup butter

Blend until light and fluffy. Chill and use when you need the sweet flavor butter.

Low-fat Pineapple Cheesecake

Here's another delicious dessert that was a hit in the classes.

Crust:

1¾ to 2 cups oat bran

½ cup pineapple juice concentrate

Mix oat bran with concentrate. Spray a pie plate with Pam and pat crust. Bake 15 min at 325° F. and set aside.

Filling:

8 ounces fat-free cream cheese

1 cup fat-free sour cream

5-6 tablespoons honey

½ cup frozen pineapple juice concentrate

½ cup evaporated skimmed milk

1 teaspoon vanilla extract

3 egg whites, unbeaten

1-10 ounce can crushed pineapple, drained

Beat cream cheese, sour cream, honey, juice concentrate, milk, vanilla and set aside. In another bowl, beat egg whites to soft peak stage. Fold into mixture and beat until well blended. Pour half of mixture into prepared crust. Spread pineapple over mixture. Top with remaining mixture. Bake at 325° F. for 60-70 minutes. Cheesecake is done when center appears set but jiggles slightly when shaken. When you remove from oven, loosen edges of cake with knife to prevent cracking. Cool for 1 hour and refrigerate for 6 hours until set. Top with fruit topping.

Fruit Topping

1-10 ounce can crushed pineapple

2 tablespoons cornstarch or arrowroot powder

1 teaspoon water

Dissolve cornstarch or arrowroot in water. Mix cornstarch or arrowroot mixture with pineapple juice mixture in a pan and bring to a boil over medium heat. Reduce heat to low and cook 5 minutes until mixture thickens. Cool. Pour glaze over cheesecake just before serving.

Holiday Orange Cranberry Bread

A wonderful tasty holiday bread.

2 cups whole-wheat pastry flour

½ cup unbleached white flour

1 tablespoon baking powder

Dash salt

1½ cups whole cranberries

1 cup orange juice

1 egg or egg replacer

¾ cup honey

½ cup fructose, sugar or Sucanat

1½ teaspoons grated orange rind

1 teaspoon vanilla

Optional: chopped walnuts

Preheat oven to 350° F. Combine flours, baking powder, and salt in a bowl. In another bowl, combine cranberries, orange juice, egg, sweeteners, grated orange rind and vanilla. Add wet ingredients to dry ingredients and stir until moistened. Batter should not be too thick, but not too thin either. Spoon into an oiled 9 x 9 inch pan and bake for 44-50 minutes.

Healthy Hermits

These are a deliciously spicy holiday cookie.

1½ cups whole-wheat pastry flour

1½ teaspoons Rumford Baking Powder

½ teaspoon each: ground allspice and cinnamon

¼ teaspoon each: ground cloves and nutmeg

¼ **cup olive or canola oil**

**1 cup Fruitsource sweetener (or Sucanat, or date
   sugar)**

2 eggs, beaten

¼ **cup apple juice**

¼ **teaspoon vanilla extract**

¼ **cup raisins**

Mix oil, Fruitsource sweetener or other sweetener, eggs or
egg replacer, apple juice and vanilla. Combine in another
bowl: flour, baking powder and spices. Add dry ingredients
to liquids and mix until well combined, but don't overmix.
Add raisins. Drop by teaspoonfuls on a cookie sheet coated
with vegetable cooking spray. Bake at 325° F. for about 20
minutes. Cool on wire rack.

Nut Butter Balls

*These are delicious, tasty and highly nutritious. Great for
a snack too.*

½ **cup nut butter (almond, peanut or sesame)**

½ **cup honey**

1 cup raisins

½ **cup dates**

2 teaspoons wheat germ

½ **teaspoon cloves**

1 teaspoon lemon or orange peel

½ **cup ground sesame seed meal**

2 cups Rice Crispie Cereal or Nutty Rice Cereal

Combine peanut butter, honey, raisins, dates and wheat
germ in a bowl, add seasonings and stir well. If you need to,

wet your hands and form into small balls. Use 2 cups Rice Crispy Brown Rice Cereal and stir gently until the cereal is well coated. Roll into ground sesame seed meal. Chill and serve. Put on a cookie sheet and freeze; then put in a zip lock bag. (You can find healthy cereals at your health food store.)

Cocoa Mini Muffins with Chocolate Chips

These are wonderfully rich and delicious. I like to bake them in a mini-muffin tin.

1 cup whole-wheat flour

½ cup cocoa powder

2½ teaspoons baking powder

¼ teaspoon salt

1 teaspoon baking soda

½ cup honey

1 cup milk

1 egg

1 cup dairy free chocolate chips (Sunspire)

Combine whole-wheat flour, cocoa, baking powder, sea salt and soda. In another bowl, combine honey, milk, and egg. Mix wet ingredients with dry ingredients. Stir in chocolate chips. Pour in oiled mini muffin tins and bake at 350° F. for 8-10 minutes.

Healthy Caramel Party Mix

1 cup soy nuts

1 cup pop corn

1 cup alphabet or waffle pretzels

1 cup Rice Checks or favorite cereal

Seasoning:

1 cup brown rice syrup

2 tablespoons molasses

¼ teaspoon salt

2 tablespoons canola oil

1 teaspoon vanilla

Combine brown rice syrup, molasses, sea salt and oil in a saucepan. Bring to a soft boil and simmer for 1-2 minutes. Stir in vanilla. Pour over mixture and stir well to coat. Transfer to a flat cookie sheet and bake at 250° F. for 20 minutes. Take out of pan and spoon into a bowl. It will harden as it cools. Cool and serve.

Gingerbread Cookies

Here is a healthy version of a Christmas favorite.

4 cups whole-wheat pastry flour

1 teaspoon baking powder

½ teaspoon ground ginger, cinnamon and cloves

¼ teaspoon salt

¼ cup Sucanat

½ cup molasses

¼ cup oil (and 3 tablespoon butter)

2 egg whites

½ cup milk

Combine dry ingredients together. In another bowl cream egg, oil, honey and molasses. Add flour alternately with milk, beating after each addition. Freeze or chill dough for one-half hour. Roll out dough and cut out cookies with a gingerbread man cookie cutter. Put on a greased cookie sheet and bake in well greased loaf pan at 350° F. for 8 to 10 minutes.

Icing:

½ cup Soyakaas cream cheese (or Neufchatel

reduced-fat cream cheese)

1 teaspoon brown rice syrup

¼ cup plus 2 teaspoons fructose

½ teaspoon vanilla extract

1 drop lemon extract

Put all ingredients in a mixing bowl and using a mixer, cream the ingredients together. This is enough frosting for an 8" square baking pan. Double the recipe to frost a two layer cake.

Variation: To make chocolate frosting, add ½ cup of WONDERSLIM cocoa powder (99.7% caffeine free.)

Absolutely No-Fat Brownies

These brownies are delicious and they contain absolutely no fat! They also have no eggs, and no cow's milk. The only fat is from optional chopped walnuts, if you want to sprinkle some on top.

1¼ cups whole wheat pastry flour

¼ teaspoon baking soda

¼ teaspoon salt

1 cup Sucanat or date sugar

1 cup cocoa powder (99.7% caffeine free) or carob

powder

5-6 tablespoons FRUITSOURCE Sweetener and

Fat Replacer

1 teaspoon vanilla

1 cup milk or soy milk

233

Optional: walnuts, chopped (or other nuts)

Preheat oven to 325° F.   Oil an 8-inch square pan. Combine flour, baking soda and salt, Sucanat and cocoa powder.   In another bowl, combine butter or fat substitute, milk, and vanilla.   Add liquid ingredients to solid ingredients and mix well.   Spread in pan and if desired, sprinkle lightly with walnuts.   Bake for 30-35 minutes or until toothpick comes out clean.   Cool and cut into squares.

Apple Crisp

6 tart apples, peeled and chopped

1 teaspoon cinnamon

¼ cup brown sugar

Topping:

½ cup 50/50 whole-wheat/unbleached white flour

¼ cup brown sugar

3 tablespoons butter

Toss the apples, cinnamon and brown sugar together in an oiled 2-quart baking dish. Set aside. Preheat an oven to 350 degrees. Make the topping by combining the flour and sugar, and then cut the butter into the flour mixture until it's crumbly. Sprinkle topping over apples and bake for about 55 -60 minutes, until slightly browned.

PART FIVE

Appendices

Healthy Cooking Techniques

Stir-fry: Commonly used in a wok, cooking food over high heat while constantly moving the food. It requires a minimum of fat and yields crisp tender foods.

Sauté: Cooking food quickly in a small amount of fat in a skillet over direct heat. Coating non-stick skillets with vegetable cooking spray is popular, or you can sauté food in a small amount of broth, wine, or water.

Poach: Cook foods in water or other liquid that is held just below the boiling point at a gentle simmer. This keeps foods moist without adding fat. Use a broth to impart flavor.

Steam: Cook foods over boiling water, normally on a stainless steel or bamboo rack with holes that allow steam to rise and cook the food. Steaming seals foods with moist heat and retains their flavor, texture and nutrients. A popular form of cooking grains, vegetables and some legumes. Adding spices to the water will infuse the food. No fat is necessary when steaming foods.

Roast: Baking at a constant moderate temperature (300° F. to 350° F.) to produce a moist interior and a well-browned exterior. Poultry and meats should be placed on a rack so they don't cook in their own drippings. Oven roast vegetables like potatoes, carrots, onions.

Broil: Food is cooked under the heat source, most commonly in an oven. Cooking temperatures are regulated by the distance between the food and heat. It's best to preheat broiler and broil 6 inches from flame. For best flavor, try marinating foods before broiling.

Grill: Food is placed on a grid above the heat source, and fat drops away from the food. The smoke produced helps flavor the food. It's commonly done outside, but modern kitchen grills are popular.

Braise: Braising is similar to stewing, only with less liquid. It means browning food and then cooking tightly covered in a small amount of liquid at a low heat for a long period of time. To braise vegetables, cut and cover with liquid. Cover the pot and place it over a low heat to prevent scorching.

Bake: Cooks food in oven with dry heat. It's similar to roasting except used for breads, casseroles, and desserts. Always bake in a pre-heated oven since the heat prevents juices from escaping from foods and drying out. For low-fat baking use a non-stick pan or a pan sprayed with vegetable oil.

Helpful Utensils

You may be aware that certain cookware is more healthy than others. I recommend that you stay away from aluminum cookware because your food will draw aluminum from the cookware. (Excess aluminum in the brain has been linked to several conditions, including Alzheimer's.) Stainless steel, enamel, glass and cast iron are better. Non-stick surfaces are okay as long as you use low heat, and don't use them if the surface is cracked or broken. Here is a short list to get you started.

Stainless steel saucepans with lids

Stainless steel wok

1 or 2 glass baking dishes

Vegetable steamer

Blender

Vegetable grater

Wooden spoons

Coffee or nut mill

Food processor

Large skillet

Colander

Cutting board

Bowl scraper

Sifter

Mixed bowl set
Measuring cups
Measuring spoons
Cutting knife

Bakeware:
Cookie sheet
Round cake pans
Square pans
Bread loafs
Pie plates
Can opener
Spatula
Potato peeler
Paring knife
Cheese grater
Wire whisk
Rolling pin

Weights and Measures

Measuring ingredients accurately is important for the proper results in cooking, but once you get the hang of it, it will be easier to master. Be careful to measure strong herbs and spices away from your cooking pot or bowl, since it's easy to accidentally add too much. I know from experience that there's no way to fix chili that has too much cayenne!

The best measuring utensils are stainless steel or glass. Most department stores or kitchen ware stores carry a nice supply. Measure liquids in a cup on a flat surface and read the desired mark at eye level. For dry ingredients, scoop or fill the cup in the individual cups and level off with a knife.

Measuring spoons come in sets of 1 tablespoon, 1 teaspoon, 1/2 teaspoon, 1/4 teaspoon and often 1/8 teaspoon. These are great for small amounts of liquids, or herbs and condiments. Dip into dry ingredients and level off with a straight edge or knife.

Liquid Measures:

3 teaspoons = 1 tablespoon = 1/2 fluid ounces

2 tablespoons = 1 fluid ounce

1 cup = 8 fluid ounces

1 cup = 1/2 pint = 8 fluid ounces

2 cups = 1 pint = 16 fluid ounces

4 cups = 1 quart = 32 fluid ounces

4 quarts = 1 gallon = 62 fluid ounces

Dry Measures:

A pinch = 1/8 teaspoon or less

2 tablespoons = 1/8 cup

3 teaspoons = 1 tablespoon

4 tablespoons = 1/4 cup

51/3 tablespoons = 1/3 cup

8 tablespoons = 1/2 cup

102/3 tablespoons = 2/3 cup

12 tablespoons = 3/4 cup

16 tablespoons = 1 cup or 1/2 pint

Oven Temperatures:

Very slow = 250°-275°

Slow = 300°-325°

Moderate = 350°-375°

Hot = 400°-425°

Very hot = 450°-475°

Extremely hot = 500°-525°

Sugar Substitutes

If you read the ingredient labels on fat-free products, you'll notice one common ingredient: white sugar! Refined white sugar is full of empty calories, contains no fiber and few nutrients. The average American eats 170 pounds of sugar per year. Eating refined white sugar causes vitamin and mineral deficiencies and weight gain. Most health-conscious consumers are opting for not only a lower fat intake, but a lower sugar intake. While all sugars should be used in moderation, some are better than others for cooking and baking.

I prefer stevia whenever possible because it doesn't affect your blood sugar level. However, for those special occasions when you want to make something healthier, here are some healthy alternatives to refined white sugar with a short conversion chart at the end. Some are available in your grocery store; others will be found in a health food store.

Barley Malt Syrup or Granules: A sweetener made from barley malt which has a naturally sweet, nutty flavor. Barley malt syrup is nice for baked goods and the granules are nice for desserts or cooking. Three-fourths cup barley malt syrup will replace one cup of sugar. Reduce the liquid by ¼ cup per one cup sugar replaced.

Brown Rice Syrup: A syrup made from brown rice which is more complex than simple sugars like honey and sugar. The syrup is not as sweet as sugar and has a delicate malt flavor. It's highly nutritious, retaining most of the nutrients found in rice. It's a good substitute for honey or liquid sweeteners when you want to decrease the sweetness of a recipe. Use ½ cup in place of one cup of sugar and reduce liquid ¼ cup.

Another type of rice syrup is Devan Sweet granulated brown rice sugar. Devan Sweet has a mild taste and lends itself well to recipes which usually require a powder rather than a liquid. Use cup-for-cup to replace white sugar.

Date Sugar: Made from dried dates which have been ground into granules, date sugar is more flavorful than sugar. However, it doesn't dissolve like white sugar, so mix it with the ingredients and let sit. It's also less dense than white sugar, so it's not as sweet. It can be substituted for white sugar cup per cup.

FruitSource: Made from white grape juice and brown rice, this commercial sweetener has a neutral flavor, although it's as sweet as white sugar. It can be found in both granular and liquid form. Three-fourths cup liquid of FruitSource replaces one cup of sugar. One and one-fourth cups of granular FruitSource will replace one cup of sugar. Mix the granules ahead and let sit before proceeding.

Frozen Fruit Juice Concentrates: Use frozen; do not let thaw first. Varieties include apple juice, orange juice, pear juice or even grape juice. Select the juice according to the recipe. For example, apple juice works nicely in carrot cake, and orange juice in orange muffins. Be sure to use the unsweetened variety. Mix your muffins quickly when you cook with fruit concentrates so that the produce will rise properly. Use one-to-one and-a-half cups of fruit juice concentrate to replace one cup of sugar and increase dry ingredients by $\frac{1}{4}$ cup. Fruit puree which means pureeing fresh fruit in a blender, also can take the place of fruit concentrates.

Fruit Sweet: Another commercial sweetener from Wax Orchards made from peach, pear and unsweetened pineapple juices. It comes in a liquid and is used like honey.

Honey: Honey be used wherever you use sugar or artificial sweeteners. Honey adds moistness and flavor to baked goods, which helps to reduce the need for much fat. Foods made with honey don't dry out as fast, and they taste even better the second and third day after baking. Honey is 20 percent sweeter than sugar, so when replacing for sugar, use less. Diabetics should use honey sparingly. To use honey in cooking, spray your measuring cup with vegetable spray and then measure the honey. It will pour out easily without any scraping. One tablespoon of honey equals 5 tablespoons of sugar. Use $\frac{3}{4}$ cup honey per 1 cup of sugar and reduce the liquid in the recipe $\frac{1}{4}$ cup.

Maple Sugar: Made from dehydrated maple syrup, it has a strong maple flavor for baked goods. Use 1 cup per 1 cup of sugar.

Maple Syrup: Boiled down sap of maple trees, maple syrup adds wonderful rich flavor to baked goods, baked beans and recipes with chocolate. The best is made without formaldehyde. Use $\frac{3}{4}$ cup per 1 cup of sugar and reduce liquid $\frac{1}{4}$ cup.

Molasses: This is pure sugarcane juice which has been boiled down to a thick syrup. The darker blackstrap molasses is strong and only requires a few tablespoons per recipe. It's nice in sweet and sour dishes too. Molasses is known to be rich in the B vitamins, iron and calcium. Use $\frac{1}{2}$ cup per cup of white sugar and if necessary, reduce the liquid by $\frac{1}{4}$ cup.

Stevia: An herb that has been approved by the FDA as a supplement, Stevia also makes a nice sweetener. Stevia is available in a dry powder form and also as a black liquid extract, so you may want to take color in consideration when you bake, since the liquid will darken your batter. Dark stevia has a almost licorice like taste. Only 1 teaspoon is required to replace 1 cup of sugar. If you use stevia in place of honey, add more liquid to make up the difference. If you use it in place of a dry sweetener like sugar or Sucanat, add dry ingredients to make up the difference.

Sucanat: One of the most popular sweeteners, Sucanat is full of vitamins and minerals and is made from evaporated sugarcane juice. Sucanat contains Vitamins A and C, calcium, iron, potassium and chromium. It has a mild taste similar to that of brown sugar and can be replaced for white sugar cup-for-cup. Sucanat Pure Cane Syrup is now available and is great for pancakes or baking.

Other sweeteners you might consider are: unsweetened apple butter, unsweetened fruit spreads or jams, and fruit juice concentrates.

For One Cup Sugar Use:	Reduce Liquid By:
Sucanat 1 cup	—
Fruitsource ½ cup	¼ cup
Devan sweet (rice sugar) ½ cup	—
Honey, ½ cup	¼ cup
Molasses ½ cup	¼ cup
Maple Syrup ½ cup	¼ cup
Date syrup 1 cup	—
Date sugar 1 cup	—
Barley malt 1¼ cups	¼ cup
Fruit juice concentrate 1½ cups	¼ cup

Since stevia is available in a liquid and powder, the conversion is somewhat different. Additionally, some of the powders vary in taste. Below I've written the conversions for two of powders that I have used. Stevita powder is not as strong as Body Ecology stevia. The liquid can be clear or dark.

Stevia Conversions

Sugar	Stevita	Body Ecology
1 cup	1 teaspoon	1 teaspoon
3/4 cup	1 teaspoon	1/4 teaspoon
1/2 cup	8 teaspoon	1/8 teaspoon
2 teaspoons	1/2 teaspoon	1/16 teaspoon
4 teaspoons	1 teaspoon	2/3 teaspoon

Herbs and Spices

Allspice: Dried whole berries which are ground and used in sweet curries, sauces, and fruits. Allspice is lso used with sweet vegetables and in cooking desserts, especially apple, pumpkin, and squash dishes. Allspice is often a blend of cloves, cinnamon and nutmeg.

Anise (Star): A seed (whole or ground) with a similar taste to licorice and used as a tea. It's nice in vegetables, salads, sauces, candy, sweet vegetables and fruits.

Basil: A somewhat sweet herb from dried leaves often used in Italian cooking. It goes well in vegetable dishes, sauces, salads, soups, and dressings. It's nice with tomatoes and eggplant dishes.

Bay Leaf: A tangy leaf commonly used in soups, stews and tomato sauces. Also used in salads, dry beans, sauces and vegetable dishes. The leaf is removed before serving.

Caraway: A crescent shaped seed popular in making rye bread. It's also nice in cabbage slaw, soups, casseroles, sauces, potatoes, green salads, and curry-rice dishes.

Cardamom: Whole seeds or ground pod, it has a lemon-ginger type flavor. It's also used in various coffee drinks, pies, and curry dishes.

Cayenne: Called the African pepper, ground cayenne pepper is hot —a little goes a long way. It's used commonly in Mexican stews, chilies and dishes. It's considered to be helpful for digestive and circulation problems. Use sparingly.

Celery Seed: A seasoning for soups, salads, sauces, stews and salad dressings.

Chervil: Dried leaves are an aromatic herb of the parsley family. It's nice in salads, sauces and soups.

Chili Powder: Blended ground chili peppers with other herbs, it's popularly used to make chili, sauces, beans and Mexican style dishes.

Chives: These leaves have an onion flavor and are nice in dips, spreads and baked potatoes. Chives belong to the onion family.

Cinnamon: Available as a bark, sticks or ground, cinnamon is a common spice used in baking, cooking and in beverages including teas, coffee and milk beverages.

Cloves: A natural breath freshener, cloves are used in cooking, and in various beverages in Indian cuisine. Cloves are used in soup, squash, yams, cider, stews and desserts.

Coriander Seed: The berry of the cilantro plant. A nutty flavor, coriander is used often in Mexican dishes. It's also used in soups, stews, vegetables, sauces and curries.

Cumin: Ground or seed, cumin has a nice spicy flavor and is used in Indian and Mexican dishes. Cumin is especially good in bean, lentil and rice dishes and is found in curries, chilies, salads, soups, and vegetables.

Curry Powder: Traditionally curry powder is a blend of various herbs often used in curry and rice dishes and often contains turmeric, cumin, coriander, cinnamon, ginger and garlic.

Dill: Dill is used frequently in Middle Eastern dishes and also with cabbage, vegetables, salads, soups, sauces, dips, dressings, spreads, pickles, cucumbers and potatoes.

Fennel Seed: The seed is similar to licorice, and is used in dressings and sauces, salads and soups.

Fenugreek: Available whole or as ground seeds, fenugreek is used in Indian curries and in Egypt as a condiment. It's popular as a tea and used in vegetables and sauces.

Garlic: Used in Italian cooking, garlic has a strong zesty flavor. Garlic has been historically used to build the immune system and lower blood pressure and cholesterol. Garlic is used in casseroles, grain dishes, salads, stews, beans and salad dressings.

Ginger: Ginger has a spicy, pungent flavor. It's used in many oriental dishes and stir fries. It's used for stomach and digestive problems, and to flavor vegetable dishes, fruit salads, bean and grain dishes.

Guaram Masala: A blend of spices which is slightly sweeter than most curry which contains no turmeric.

Licorice: Licorice has a similar taste to anise, and is frequently used to make licorice candy. It may help with cravings for sweets.

Mace: Mace comes from the covering of nutmeg, and is used popularly in baking and cooking. It's nice in cakes, desserts, fruit salads, sauces and curries.

Marjoram: Marjoram is available ground or as whole leaves. Part of the mint family, marjoram is used in Italian dishes and also in soups, stews, dressings stuffing, and salads.

Mint and Peppermint: Both have a fresh taste which is often good for digestion. Both are nice with fruit or vegetable dishes, sauces, dips and dressings. They blend well with other herbs and are nice in fruit punches, beverages, mint sauces, tea and in the popular Taboulie salad.

Mustard: Black mustard seeds are popular in Indian dishes. Yellow mustard seeds are used in relishes, curries and salads, cabbage dishes and spreads.

Nutmeg: Available as ground or whole seeds, nutmeg is popularly used in baking sweet desserts, soups, sauces and fruit dishes.

Onion: Found in the garlic family, onions are used to flavor foods from around the world. Onion, garlic, scallions and chives are all related herbs of the lily family.

Oregano: Available as ground or dried, whole leaves, oregano is used in Greek, Italian, French and Mexican dishes. It's also in the mint family. Use small amounts, as it can overpower other herbs. It's nice in sauces, salad dressings, pizza, spaghetti sauce, and vegetable dishes.

Paprika: A mild, sweet pepper, paprika is nice in casseroles, soups, potatoes, salad dressings, sauces and vegetables.

Parsley: A bitter green herb used as a garnish, parsley is very high in chlorophyll and minerals. It's nice in salads, salad dressings, rice pilaf and as a flavoring for dips, soups, sauces and pasta.

Poppy Seed: Used in dressings, sauces, salads, vegetables, and grain dishes, poppy seeds are used as a topping for breads and cookies.

Rosemary: Rosemary has somewhat of a pine taste. It's used in combination with other herbs for salad dressings and tomato sauces.

Saffron: Often used in rice dishes, saffron adds a golden color to many dishes; used in Indian cooking.

Sage: Another aromatic herb, sage is nice in soups, sauces and dressings. A member of the mint family, it's nice in stuffings, soup, beans, vegetables, rice dishes and curries.

Savory: Used as whole and ground leaves, savory has a mild peppery flavor. It's also nice in salads, soups, sauces and dressings and works well with thyme and marjoram.

Sesame Seeds: The seeds of a tropical herbal plant, sesame seeds are used in baking, and as a garnish for breads and casseroles and in green bean, rice and stir-frys.

Tarragon: Available whole and as ground dried leaves, tarragon is used in dressings, salads, sauces, casseroles, soups, fruits, tomato based dishes, broccoli and curries.

Thyme: Thyme leaves are dried and ground and popularly used in poultry stuffings and salad dressings, stews, soups, split peas, lentils, onions, peas, carrots, and green beans.

Turmeric: Used in Indian dishes, curries and rice dishes, tumeric adds yellow color to dishes and is used in salads, sauces, vegetables, rice and soups.

Vanilla: Vanilla is used in whole bean form or as extract. It's popular in baked good, puddings, nuts milks, and sweet sauces.

Appendix F

Beans

Aduki or Azuki: Small red Japanese beans which are quick cooking, easy to digest and somewhat sweet. Said to be good food for the kidneys, they are nice when cooked with brown rice or sprouted and used in salads.

Anasaki: Ancestor of the pinto beans, these cook faster than pintos and lend themselves to Mexican dishes with garlic and chili. They have a rich, somewhat sweet flavor.

Black Beans: Also called Turtle beans, these are a staple of Latin American, Asian and Cuban diets. They blend well with corn, rice and spices. Versatile, they can be made in soups, spreads, salads and burgers. Black beans are a great source of protein and fiber.

Black-eyed peas: Also known as cowpeas, these thin skinned peas are popular in Southeastern United States, India and Africa. Quick cooking, they make good soups, stuffings and casseroles. They are especially good with corn bread and rice.

Fava Beans: Flat kidney shaped beans, fava beans are often used in soups with pasta. The outer skin is tough, so these are peeled after cooking.

Garbanzo beans: Also known as Chick-peas, these are small, round dried legumes tan in color. Used often mashed in Middle Eastern dishes like Humus and Indian dishes, these beans are high in calcium and are delicious in dips, curries, soups, salads, casseroles and burgers. They have a mildly nutty flavor.

Great Northern Beans: Also called white beans, these make delicious baked beans. Navy beans are somewhat smaller white beans which take a little longer to cook. These beans are mild in flavor and are also nice in soups or stews.

Kidney beans: Also called red kidney beans, these beans have a distinct rich flavor and are best known in chili recipes. They are fast cooking and hold their shape well.

Lentils: Flat, round legumes which come in reddish-orange, green colors, lentils are delicious with a somewhat peppery flavor. Quick-cooking they are especially nice in curry dishes, soups and stews.

Lima Beans: When soaked lima beans cook fairly quickly, but be sure not to overcook or they will get mushy. Otherwise, they are nice in soups, salads or casseroles. They are used frequently in Central and South America, have a buttery flavor. They make a great side dish.

Mung Beans: A small round green bean, also easy to cook and frequently sprouted as in Chinese bean sprouts. They are used in Indian curry dishes and Indian dahls. Mung bean pasta also known as mung bean threads is available in Asian markets.

Navy Beans: See Great Northern.

Pinto Beans: Plump, pinkish brown flecked beans, pinto beans are often spiced with garlic, chilies and cumin, and are often used in Mexican dishes like bean dips and bean burritos.

Red Beans: See kidney beans.

Soy beans: A versatile bean which is high in protein, lecithin and the good type of Omega 3 fatty acids. Soy products include: tofu, tempeh, soy sauce, miso, TVP (texturized vegetable protein), soy milk, soy cheese, soy cream cheese, soy yogurt, soy oil, soy nuts and soy flour. These beans can also be sprouted for salads. (See Tofu and Tempeh section for more information.)

Split peas: These are yellow and green peas in the lentil family. Since these are skinless, they need no soaking and tend to dissolve when cooked. Their mild flavor makes a nice soup with herbs like thyme and rosemary. Green split peas are common in split pea soup.

Appendix G

Grains

Amaranth: An ancient grain, similar to sesame seeds which was cultivated and highly prized by the Aztecs and Chinese. A high quality gluten-free protein, amaranth is high in the amino acid lysine. You might want to use it with other grains, since it cooks up like a glutinous porridge. Add it to soups, casseroles, breads and even muffins or cookies for added protein. Amaranth flour is a great nutritional boost to baked goods. Or, leftover amaranth can be sautéed in butter for a delicious breakfast cereal. Amaranth has a gelitenous quality and a somewhat nutty flavor. This grain can be popped like corn.

Barley: Barley is a low-gluten grain used to make barley flour and barley malt syrup, (a mild sweetener used for baking cookies and muffins). A popular grain in North Africa and South East Asia, barley is often used as a cereal and to thicken soups or stews. Hulled whole barley, the most nutritious also takes the longest to cook, even when soaked. Pearled barley is another name for polished barley which is quick cooking, but not as nutritious. Lightly pearled, semi-hulled barley is the most nutritious. Barley is used to make barley miso and barley malt for brewing beer, and malted milkshakes. Barley can be made into a flour (ground groats), or as grits, pearled, sprouts, or malted.

Buckwheat: A non-wheat seed high in nutritional value and often used in cold climates, buckwheat is said to be a blood builder. Buckwheat is high in protein, minerals, vitamins and enzymes if sprouted. It's used traditionally in buckwheat pancakes. Kasha is a Russian staple made from cooked buckwheat. White buckwheat groats make a milder buckwheat flour than regular buckwheat groats. Soba buckwheat noodles are delicious noodles found in many Japanese dishes and are a great way to enjoy this hearty grain. Buckwheat can be sprouted, toasted, made into grits, flour, or noodles.

Corn: Sweet corn is eaten as a vegetable. Field corn is often called maize and is available as popcorn, grits, hominy, corn meal, masa harina and blue corn. Corn grits (polenta) are coarsely ground cornmeal, or hulled kernels of dried white or yellow corn. Corn grits make a great breakfast food, cooked like other cereal grains. After it's cooled, polenta is often cooled, sliced and sautéed in butter or oil, a popular dish in Northern Italy. I've used polenta to make a nice crust for Mexican casseroles. Blue corn has 21 percent more protein and more minerals than other corns and is used often to make delicious blue corn chips. I don't recommend "degermed" corn meal because much of the hull and nutritional value has been removed. Whole grain corn meal, soaked in lime water is called masa harina and used in Latin America for making tortillas. Corn can be made into corn meal, corn flour, corn grits, flaked, hominy, pop corn, corn starch, tortillas, corn bran. Hominy is polished white or yellow corn soaked in lye solution or lime to soften the hull and swell the grains. Hominy is available canned, dried or frozen.

Kamut: Kamut, the Egyptian name for wheat is a type of durhum wheat, very high in protein and other minerals. When they refer to Roman granaries in Cleopatra's time, the wheat they ate was kamut. A rice-like grain, kamut triples in volume when cooked and is nice mixed with rice. I really enjoy the pasta made from kamut which is mild tasting yet high in nutrition. Kamut is also available as a flour, but may be hard to find as a whole grain.

Millet: A staple of Egypt, Asia and North Africa, millet is a gluten-free grain rich in amino acids and alkalizing to the stomach. Millet looks like tiny round yellow kernels often used in a birdseed mixture in the United States. Good for people with wheat allergies or candida, millet is often used interchangeably with rice. Millet also makes a good cooked cereal, main dish or salad or can be used to thicken soups or sauces. With a nice mild, nutty flavor, millet can be made into flour, meal, cracked or sprouts.

Oats: Oats are a whole grain eaten frequently in Britain, Scotland and Northern Europe. A great replacement for wheat. Oats are an excellent source of fiber which helps to lower cholesterol and promote regularity. Oats are available rolled, flaked, steel cut and used as a thickening agent, or in baked goods, casseroles, pancakes, etc. Oat bran contains a valuable high soluble fiber.

Oat groats refer to the whole grain. Steel cut oats are coarser and often called "Irish oatmeal." The quick cooking oats are often broken into smaller pieces. I like using oat flour as an added flour in desserts and pie crusts since it has a slightly sweet flavor.

Oats are available as whole, rolled, steel cut, oat flakes, oatmeal, oat milk, oat sprouts, oat flour and oat bran.

Quinoa (keen-wa): A tiny grain no bigger than a mustard seed, quinoa once fed an ancient civilization. Called a supergrain and highly prized by the Incas, quinoa is a high-quality, complete protein grain rich in vitamins E, B and minerals. Quinoa looks like a cross between sesame seeds and millet. Fairly quick cooking, quinoa contains more protein than all other grains and is high in lysine. Use quinoa like rice or millet. It's also gluten free.

Rice: Eaten often in China, India and Southeast Asia, rice is the second most produced food in the world. Brown rice is the most nutritional of the rice family, high in B vitamins and vitamin E. White rice is brown rice that was polished to remove the bran and germ, so it's not as nutritious as brown rice. If you follow my cooking instructions, you can come out with a delicious rice that your family will enjoy.

Long grain: Dry and fluffy, and nice for people who are used to white rice.

Medium grain: Short, moist grains, this rice grows in California, Spain and Italy.

Short grain: Soft and somewhat sticky, short-grain rice makes a nice rice pudding and stuffings. Short brown rice is my favorite since it's chewy and nutritious. It takes about 50-55 minutes to cook.

Sweet brown rice: A glutinous rice, sweet brown rice is especially nice for desserts. Pounded sweet brown rice, called Mochi is particularly good for people with weak digestion.

Special rices: There are hundreds of varieties of rice. Here a few common ones:

Basmati Rice: Another type of whole-grain rice from India and Pakistan. It's better than white rice and ligher and easier to digest than brown rice. It's fairly quick cooking and has a wonderful aroma when cooking.

Texmati Rice: A hybrid of Indian basmati and long-grain American rice, this rice has a popcorn aroma and somewhat nutty taste. Quick-cooking, Texmati rice cooks in 25 minutes, and results in fluffy grains.

Wehani: A rice developed by pioneers from California who formed the Lundberg company. A rust colored rice, wehani cooks like rice and tastes similar to chestnuts. Another type of rice created by the Lundberg brothers is Riz Cous, which resembles couscous. Riz Cous is a cracked rice, which is used interchangeably with couscous.

Wild Rice: Wild rice is not really a cereal grain. Wild rice is delicious, high in fiber and low in calories. Many varieties are available, especially in health food stores and specialty stores. Most wild rice cooks in 45-60 minutes and is especially nice mixed with equal parts of brown rice.

Rye berries: Rye is a staple grain of Europe and Russia which resembles wheat but has a distinctly different taste. Rye comes in whole, cracked and flaked forms. Flaked rye is often used in granola. Rye is commonly used ground for flour in rye bread, or cooked as a cereal.

Spelt: An ancient relative of the wheat family, spelt is another high protein grain that has been "rediscovered." A biblical reference to spelt is found in Ezekiel 4:9. It is related to wheat, with a sweet, nutty taste. Spelt contains gluten but is easier to digest than wheat. Popular in Europe, spelt is used in soups and stews. Spelt is a hearty grain which needs to be soaked before cooking. Many people who are allergic to wheat can eat spelt. Spelt is made into pasta, breads cereals and flour. Spelt is higher in protein than wheat and lower in gluten.

Triticale: A hybrid of wheat and rye berries which contains adequate gluten for bread baking. Especially nice as a flour for bread baking, triticale is slightly higher in protein than wheat, and low in gluten.

Wheat Kernels: The most widely-used cereal in the world, grown nearly in every country, wheat berries are the whole-wheat kernel complete with the germ and bran. Wheat berries are used as a cereal, or ground into flour for baking muffins, breads, and other desserts. Sprouted wheat berries are a great addition to breads. Manna bread is a type of bread made entirely from sprouted wheat kernels. Wheat Germ is the seed or germ of the kernel, often sold as a source of vitamin E and other minerals. Wheat bran has been sold separately, also but is not as good a fiber source as oat bran. Hard wheat contains high levels of protein while soft wheat contains more carbohydrates. Types of wheat are cracked wheat, durum wheat (for pasta) and kamut (a durum wheat with 40% more protein.) Parts of wheat are wheat germ, wheat bran, whole wheat flour and whole wheat pasta, cracked and bulgur wheat.

Wheat Bran: The outer layer of a kernel of grain, usually processed out of refined grains as with white flour. The bran contains most of the B vitamins, minerals and fibers. Oat, rice and wheat bran are available, although wheat bran is too hard for most people's digestive tract.

Wheat Germ: This is the seed of a grain which contains valuable nutrients like protein, minerals and vitamins including vitamin E. Wheat germ is commonly sold separately as in wheat and corn germ which are highly perishable and need to be kept in a tightly sealed container in the refrigerator. Wheat germ is a nice addition to casseroles and loaves and has a nutty like flavor.

Couscous: is cracked and partially cooked wheat which is a lighter fluffier texture made from semolina wheat which has been precooked before it's dried.

Cracked Wheat: is grain cracked into coarse pieces with the bran and germ left. Cracked wheat is uncooked wheat berries so it must be boiled in water before eating. A coarse ground cracked wheat would be suited for Taboulie or a pilaf.

Bulgur: is a cooked, steamed and dried wheat which cooks in 5-10 minutes. Bulgur is traditionally used in the Middle East salad called Taboulie, made with bulgur, tomatoes, parsley, lemon juice, olive oil and spices. Hard wheat has more protein and soft wheat has more carbohydrates. It's often used in place of couscous, or ground nuts and is available in fine, medium or coarse ground.

Recipe Index

PARTY BEVERAGES AND DESSERTS

Subject Index

U-V

Utensils, 238
Vanilla, 249
Vegetables, 124
Vegetable Entrees, 124
Vegetarian, 165
Vinegars, 108
Vinaigrette Dressing, 112

W

Waldorf Salad, 122
Weights and Measures, 240
Wheat, 30, 52, 55, 204
White Sauce, 107
Whole Wheat Bread, 204
White Bean Chili, 154

XYZ

Yogurt, 214
Zucchini, 96